*To a have a of peace, happy Mica, Love Always, Jan*

We are light returning to light.
Most valuable, is experiencing our every breath
as a reminder we do belong here at this time—
to love and be loved.
May we clear away all that no longer shines,
exhale it, and breathe life into the shadows
of our beautiful souls—separation and lack illusions,
evaporating back into nothingness!
May we all be blessed with the beauty way
of giving light and not heat.
May we all have the strength and self-love to explore
inflammation and it's root causes.
May all sentient beings be happy and free!

# EarthGut

Story of
## *PEACE, LOVE & MICROBES*

Tami S. Hay RMT, MA.

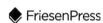 FriesenPress

Suite 300 - 990 Fort St
Victoria, BC, V8V 3K2
Canada

www.friesenpress.com

ISBN
978-1-5255-5330-1 (Hardcover)
978-1-5255-5331-8 (Paperback)
978-1-5255-5332-5 (eBook)

*1. HEALTH & FITNESS, HEALING*

Distributed to the trade by The Ingram Book Company

## *Acknowledgements of Deep Gratitude:*

To my teachers and mentors: Dr. Rabbi Gabriel Cousens, Cyndi Dodick, Biologist John Phillips, and my Essene community at the Tree of Life—circles of ancestral remembrance.

A deep, heartfelt thanks to the brilliant Dr. Zach Bush and team, and all their divinely guided, heart-centred knowledge.

To Rameen and Teachers at Sattva Yoga Edmonton, much gratitude for the reflection of insight, truth and compassion. What a blessing to live in community together.

To my teachers at Hippocrates Health Institute and Optimum Health Institute: Thank you for holding healing space. And to all committees of responsible physicians everywhere!

To all my clients and soul friends, who I am so blessed to say have shared reciprocal love and teachings and have loved me home!

To my dear editor Barry who patiently guides me.

To my book designer and dear friend Pete, thank you for reciprocal kindness and enduring my ever-changing flow.

To my beloved friend Perry, who stood by me with encouragement and his computer skills, making the soul urging of this book and my Masters studies, a mindful practice. I wish you peace.

To the Creator, who is the strength of this year, and the Angels here and across the veil.

To my late son Ryan, who fuels me from across the veil after his passing in 2017. Thank you for all the teaching and holding me to the fire of authenticity.

To my beautiful daughters Jennifer and Kaitlyn whose enduring strength and love remind me of humility, sovereignty, and the abundance in family ties.

To my furry family who remind me that the love of one is the love of all.

To my grandchildren Emerlee, Phoenix, and Hadley. Thank you for playing with me, wild and free! May you be the change towards planetary reconnection into the microbial threads of ancestral truth.
May you be way-showers for the next seven generations unseen.

Much gratitude to FriesenPress and all their dedicated talented team.

### And to sacred Mother Earth, who keeps lending her microbial forgiveness.

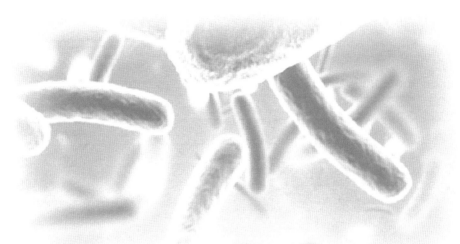

Consciousness sleeps in minerals,
it dreams in microbes and plants,
it starts to wake up in humans.

Then in some humans it says, who am I?
What's going on?

And ends up concluding the total
universe of expression.

~ *Rumi*

# Contents

## Disclaimer:

The information in this book is true and complete to the best of my knowledge and represents my personal story and self-healing. This book is intended only as an informative guide, an inspirational story for those wishing to know more about health issues, gut health and natural hygiene. In no way is this book intended to replace, countermand, or conflict with the advice given to you by your own physician and health team. The ultimate decision concerning care should be made between you and your doctors. We, the author and doctors mentioned throughout, strongly recommend you follow their advice. Information in this book is general and offered with no guarantees on the part of the authors or FriesenPress. The author and publisher disclaim all liability in connection with the use of this book.

# THE INVITATION

*You are an honored guest here*
*At this feast called life*
*Every breath you breathe is proof*
*You belong here at this time*

*Come take this place set for you*
*And choose each dish with clear intention*
*For each will lead you in a different direction*
*And perhaps enough dishes have been servings of suffering*

*It is all self-serve from here*
*So choose the "light" menu*
*For it is time to walk*
*With light-hearted ease down your path*

*Enjoy the journey*
*For you are but a guest here*
*For a very short while*
*And you were never meant to leave this world*
*Carrying a sack of regrets*

*Spend time each day with the silence of your inner flame*
*For the wise ones dwell there*
*Seek their counsel often*
*For you are wiser than you know*

*And from that fork in the road*
*You will always find the path*
*Leading you back home*
*To your honored place*
*At our table.*

# My Story:

# *Making the Connection*

*We are not our story. We are much greater than our story.*
*Yet our story may light our path into a wellspring of awakening.*

In 2006 I was diagnosed with ulcerative colitis, an inflammatory
bowel disease (IBD), which I thought was a two-month flu affecting my
digestive system. The next three years saw me in and out of hospital,
severely dehydrated, with bouts of medication only relieving symptoms
for a short while and did not heal. The final diagnosis of Crohn's (because
of the multi-layers of musculature lining that were damaged) including
fistulation. An intensely inflamed bowel takes us out fast!

The GI doctor on call that day told me I might need to be on antibiotics
off and on for the rest of my life to keep the fistulas from getting infected.
I knew the systemic gut damage that antibiotics did to me as a child. I had
constant ear infections which I later discovered was a severe dairy allergy.
I was so ill at the time, but I remember thinking, no way!

I found myself seeking out holistic options, ending up at Hippocrates
Health Institute at West Palm Beach, FL for their 21-day transformational
program consisting of a live food, high-chlorophyll, organic vegan diet,
juices, wheatgrass, along with various mindbody detoxification therapies

and an educational program. On my way to Hippocrates, I was so weak I could not walk along the beach. Miraculous healing after 21 days allowed me to run the beach for thirty minutes, bask in my body's renewal, and feel hope!

If you are reading this in your search for answers for healing, you will know intimately what I mean … when you begin feeling really healthy again, when hope is restored!

The bleeding in my intestines that had been present off and on for a year subsided in just two days on juicing and bowel rest. This is our body's amazing self-healing gifts! Why did this have such amazing results? It was because every single person I encountered knew; not believed but knew. I could heal and held space for my entrance into wellness. I walked through that veil into what Joe Dispenza calls my genius.

I continued to study live food, juicing and plant-based healing, and the power of rewiring my brain into infinite healing possibilities, with much success over the next 10 years. Yet this was not without challenge and many a "getting-back-on-track" days, self-inquiry and unwinding many moons of ancestral food habit, is certainly a journey!

I divinely landed at the Tree of Life Rejuvenation Centre with Dr. Gabriel Cousens and the Essenes. It is here where I finished a Masters, in Plant Based Spiritual Nutrition.

Later I was blessed with a deeper self inquiry at the Sattva School of Yoga with Rameen and into "science of self" and continued into compassionate inquiry of the biology of "true self", within the spirited brilliance of Dr. Zach Bush.[1]

Yet always a student, humbly breathing my way through this thing called wellness, I come before you here to share some learning I have deemed helpful along the way. For "I have walked a thousand miles in your moccasins" and it is from this place of heart-centred understanding I share my simple story. It is not an A to B story; it is more a spiral one with exit and entrance points of good and not-so-good choices, sadness, and joy in the ebb and flow of this miraculous thing called life. Caroline Myss once said these words of wisdom: *"We must make the decision to share our wisdom from our suffering and choose wisdom over woe!"*

It was through pain, my heart surrendered and through sweet surrender, one morning on my bathroom floor I felt such a deep presence of light, I knew I would be well and share this remembrance journey of pain transmutation into the sacred.

Since beginning this book my eldest and only son died, grandchildren were born, and I experienced many other comings and goings of life and death, grief and gratitude. Yet I was still breathing, one breath at a time. Sometimes a deep breath would get stuck in my chest, cleansing tears and longing would come, then pass, return and then, very slowly, pass again. I would sometimes indulge in food that I knew was not so helpful… and the world kept turning.

My wish for all readers and searchers of a road less travelled is to know that you truly do belong here at this time, and there are true, tested ways to freedom, wellness and pain relief—peace and ease. The gut, as it begins to remember its innate intelligence, is a self-healing organ by design; the bowel lining regenerates every 72 hours, what a miracle! I believe we all have a deep well of strength, health and goodness as long as we are breathing.

I wish for you to explore deeper possibilities within natural laws of wellness and sustainable practices. I hold for you, ease and flow.

**We are not our story. We are much vaster and greater than our story, yet our story may light the path home.**

On my lifelong journey, I have had mostly easy access to optimism and joy. Yet something happened after I was inflamed with IBD, as "dying" visited me intensely until I was left wondering whether or not I would live, or even if I wanted to. I found the easy access I once had to happiness was significantly compromised when the intestines were inflamed. I have come to understand the effects on the gut (our second brain or lost organ as many refer to it), makes up to 90% of our serotonin and 50% of our dopamine (our feel-good hormones), and it is our largest warehouse of immunity. Happiness is much less accessible when we have limited serotonin, dopamine production and GABA due to acute inflammation in the gut. This may be the root of depression and addiction for many, for we are ease-seeking beings by design. Be gentle with yourself as you find your way, for a peaceful transition is the point.

In first undertaking the challenge to heal Crohn's disease without pharmaceuticals, I began to feel the inflammation settle down while resting my bowels, heart, and mind for three weeks at a live food rejuvenation centre. The C-reactive protein (CRP) blood work test confirmed my numbers had dropped from 18–21 mg/L to 2 mg/L CRP. Between 1–2.9 mg/L shows relatively intermittent range and >10 mg/L indicates extreme inflammatory disease.

**Light, pure food, fasting and love—major components of healing!**

I do understand that everyone with IBD, in the acute stages, is recommended to never eat raw fibre. Therefore, I had relied heavily on raw pure vegetable juices (pulp removed) of high nutritional value, which assisted in the healing—along with soft fruit and raw vegetable juice smoothies (more of this in diet and bowel rest, and fasting). Knowing the bowel lining regenerates itself quickly, we can be gentle, yet still eat healing and highly enzymatic foods. This book does not lay out specific diet or lifestyle shifts for all, for that is individual by design. You can do a Viome test to know exactly what your individual dietary needs are and precise gut microbial assistance you require.

Yet, one thing is clear and well understood in integrative medicine—inflammatory substances and toxins need to be released before bowel rest and regeneration can occur, and the microbiome and beneficial bacteria restored.

This investigation and journey towards finding a diet and lifestyle that would allow me to live in remission became a multidimensional search. It landed in a plant-based, quiet life of heart healing, mostly a raw rainbow of veganic/organic food, plentiful amounts of green juice, plant-based nutrition, meditation, and the release of all that no longer serves my well-being, including people, places and distractions.

Most doctors are taught to often rely on autoimmune suppressant medication only. Knowing this, it is the individual's responsibility to do research, and there are plentiful case histories of physicians and wellness seekers who teach traditional and nutritionally sound, grounded ways to keep illness in remission or heal completely. I am not against pharmaceuticals. I am wise enough to know that what we fight or what we "force" against, will have an equal or greater push-back. Yet knowing the body makes 100,000 chemicals per second on average, we begin to understand our body is the best pharmacy we have, if we assist it. What I am passionate to bring into the equation is **balance**. The imbalance in the modern medical protocol for most disease, IBD and IBS is this: pharmaceuticals are the ONLY protocol offered to patients nearly 100% of the time.

This is not a linear path we are on. We will probably begin emotionally eating comfort food again, slump down a little. I know my way home and the cost of health is not worth the cost of pain and discomfort avoidance.

The only way through pain is through it! I know this to be true. After my son passed and I emotionally ate for a year off and on; I revisited inflammatory responses such as rashes, fatigue, mood imbalances and bowel flares-ups from gluten, sugar, and other stuff. I reset with a short fast, yoga, meditation, and life coaching from an invaluable Biology Basecamp course with Dr. Zach Bush.[1]

I furthered home-coming healing with barefoot running and walking, forest bathing and the daily cold plunges my Finnish ancestors used as the "cure" for everything, with much success. The literal translation for the Finnish word Sisu, (a word used to represent strength of mindbody), is to have guts.

I gathered my support from heaven and earth. I share this as a gentle reminder to find ease in this human experience and to understand that the longer a food trigger is out of our body, the more we will react when it is re-introduced. By being kind to ourself, home will shine us back much quicker.

I would invite you to still open yourself to the journey of this book, even if you are not yet ready to look at releasing animal products as a lifestyle, or if you have been told by physicians to never again eat raw plant fibre or that full healing is impossible. I am not giving medical advice—simply sharing a very long story and science that I have deemed helpful. This is much more of an invitation—an invitation to see and feel how a diet of health and mindfulness through breathing and re-connective healing, can change biology and restore hope and happiness!

# SWEET SURRENDER

In the endless details of doing
My heart gives away
In the moment of surrender
I was able to hear her say
You are not a human-doing
You're a human-being
And no amount of accomplishment
Justifies your worth on this Earth

For you are so valued
Simply because
you were born.

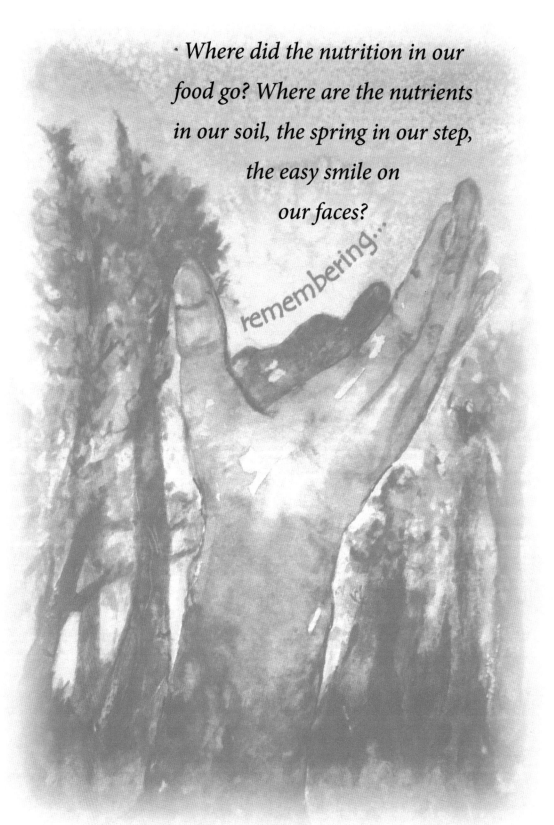

*Where did the nutrition in our food go? Where are the nutrients in our soil, the spring in our step, the easy smile on our faces?*

remembering...

# Introduction:

# A Preface of Peace, Love & Microbes

We are ONE! In understanding our interconnection, we may find a poetic place far beyond individual human chaos. It is a beautiful sacred place, where the rivers of peace, love and microbes meet Heaven on Earth. Heaven on Earth you may wonder… in a world where disharmony and disease are increasing at alarming rates? Yet what if that too, was here for our full awakening?

Still awaiting our return, is spaciousness beyond escalating illness, suffering, and chaos manifesting as separation. Nature knows no separation and what appears chaos to humans, is natural in the living world. For example, if we poured the same poison on our plants we eat and drink, naturally they would wither, go dormant, give us a couple more chances to clean up the nutrient source, and if this did not happen, it would be natural to die.

Within the very next breath, one may access insight into their true nature, and begin the journey of "the science of self," as yoga teacher Rameen Peyrow gently teaches us. Here we begin to remove the dams, (and the damns) and let the rivers flow into our natural healing abilities, integrating the *know*-how-do! It is here we may cry out, "There must be more to this story!"

In this sitting, asking, and seeking, we may understand healing as a gift of awakening—to deepen into one's true and authentic self. It is here we begin to understand that we are exposed to hundreds of times more human-created toxins and electromagnetic force, (disrupting our cellular brilliance) than ever seen in human history and in order to remain well, we must develop awareness, through some of the tools laid out before you—moving towards seeds of change.

Health issues slow us down and sometimes force us to unplug. As painful as this can be, illness has within it, the opportunist potential of gift-giving, when allowed to teach us what is no longer working. It is in this exact place we may regather our energy and fine-tune where we will allow our attention to be pulled. From heart disease to unhappiness and no-ease, the opportunity arises for another journey. The Chinese character for "crisis" means both problem and opportunity. Many people are changed in crisis. Illness has been a catalyst for human change, as it was for myself, and seeing crisis as both a problem and opportunity is essential if we are to have a felt sense of peace, love and healing microbes. In these precarious times, I am still here learning, as long as I am breathing.

**If we can truly move from the fear of illness to "being right here with what is," while imagining ourselves as well and free, we just might be able to create it!**

There is an understanding in integrative medicine: all disease begins with gut inflammation/dysbiosis and missing healing microbes. The gut brings the mind along for the ride through its vagal nerve connection. Exploring root causes of disease is so very complex yet very simple. We do know that by healing the gut through nutrition and reconnection, the mindbody may be able to regain clear health options. This book focuses on digestive disorders simply because no one who is ill has a healthy gut. This book is for everyone who does not feel energized most of the time, does not feel in flow and ease. The stories I share of healing from bowel disease, are not much different than anyone who is unwell, simply a different diagnosis, yet root causes similar; stress, disconnect, and inflammation.

Visionary Barbara Hubbard Marx would ask: "What is the role of 'crisis' in evolution? It means we cannot go back to doing the same thing!" This is true on both an individual health level and on a global level as well. So where do we begin? We begin with: "us being the change"; the medicine wheel returning to a balance of peace, love and microbes; and finding and maintaining health on a planet struggling with toxic overload. It begins with us regaining hope, one self-loving action at a time … accountable actions as stewards of Mother Earth and ALL life. This, in turn, will translate into healing the integrity of our EarthGut. EarthGut, as coined in this book, recognizes our grace and interconnection within the earth we eat from, live on, praise or poison, and how directly this translates into either a diverse thriving body and belly or a sickly mono-culture one, prone to leaks and disease. We may choose a life of pain-free ease and easy access to compassion, or quite the opposite.

We are an interwoven web of connecting microbes, and as we cultivate mindfulness—for ourselves, each other, animals, and the planet—we have a felt sense of this. We are not solid matter, we are dynamic and ever-changing water, energy, bacteria, and light. There is a microbial mystery calling us home. This biodynamic us is quite miraculously self-healing by design—a symbiosis of wonder! Yet many of us feel far removed from deep peace and ease. Ancient microbial mystery is calling us back into peace, through reestablishing our gut intelligence, balance, and higher self. When inviting **mindbody** healing into the equation, (as coined by Dr. Candace Pert in the 80s with much controversy), we may begin exploring a whole new world. When we understand ourselves and our mindbody as ONE, we can invite the following into manifestation, and find our way out of stress and dis-ease:

> **Peace**—a calm and ease-filled being.
> **Love**—self-love made manifest and shared in service within a loving Universe.
> **Our Microbiome**—collection of bacteria, fungus, virus, and yeast within the large community of immunity within our gut; when nurtured, enriched with potential life force and worthy of attention, nutrition and care.

Allowing all our actions to be ones that create a peaceful and microbial rich planet for ALL; within the consumption of REAL food and sustainable earthing practices, is a reclamation into wisdom, and freedom. It is within our inner ecology—our EarthGut—that we can begin a deeper experience of our lives.

The Buddha informed us from a special little Bodhi tree many moons ago, *"There were only two things that create suffering; the belief that we are not enough, and that we are separate."* It is within this concept of separation, that wellness falls away, stress and stagnation accumulate, and we struggle. It is only when we believe we are not in this together that we partake in destruction.

Integrative physicians and dedicated teachers of whole-person healing help us connect with the first protocol for health—nutrition of body and mind.

# *Evolve or Dissolve*

Knowing we belong here is possible when we answer the call to evolve, to create cellular hydration and a fully intact intestinal structure. It is here we can silence the chaos long enough to hear God's urging, and visualize and practice—with deep focus—a thriving self. By listening, we may be able to reclaim our birthright towards health, despite the ever-growing incidence of disease. I have come to understand our inflamed gut is Mother Earth's mirroring, revealing her compassionate guidance to detoxify. At this time in our evolution, the ratio of injury outweighs repair and we are, as humans, on the brink of … ?

Health allows us the sovereignty to respect natural laws. Sovereignty is our ability to unplug from status quo and "not true belief systems" we hold, and begin to let go.

When we destroy or manipulate our natural resources away from healthy living soil/earth diversity, it will in turn destroy our healthy gut, brain, body and our birthright to continue to evolve as pure souls. In the depths of acute inflammation, the journey to complete recovery may feel impossible. Yet, as the resurrective medicine of the hummingbird (infused on the front cover) shares, the long, seemingly impossible journey is incredibly rich with transformation when derived in the present moment. Focusing on our birthright of value and love ability, and then taking actions which integrate this truth, allows us to navigate our divine direction. Hummingbird opens the heart, a calling in these times of planetary-brink-of-destruction crisis, sprinkling the possibilities of a more heart-centred and richer way of living.

This global gathering asks us to shake free the shackles of disease identity and the conventional belief that we are powerless over illness and that our lives have become unmanageable.

"There are only two reasons we have obsessive thoughts. One is they are showing us what needs healing. The other is there is something which requires action. Either way, we need to pay attention and get to know them."

~ Rameen Peyrow

# Silencing the Inner Critic

We have 60,000-80,000 thoughts a day and 90% are the same. Which thoughts do we want to continue repeating and which do we want to begin deleting? Can we change our actions and our way of thinking as we remodel a thriving world?

In silence and body inquiry, coming home to body awareness is as quick as three belly breaths. **In getting out of future fears and into our bodies, we realize an unfocused and inflamed mind is seldom our friend.** This unkind mind will often focus on what is wrong over what is right and, believe me, no matter how ill we are, there are sparks of unbroken essence waiting without judgement to assist us toward better health!

In deeply exploring our emotional attachment to addictive comfort food and thought, we may compassionately unravel our emotional dependencies in using food as a drug to take the edge off of life. When the pseudo-security of old patterning is no longer working for us, we are at a crossroads. From here, we may begin to learn to trust our hearts, get out of our heads, and into the self-inquiring found when simply bringing stillness to our meditation butt … "no buts" …

Shakespeare was known to have said, "First, know thyself." In the silence we reunite. In self-inquiry we find many answers. When we move beyond the initial discomfort of deeply listening, we begin to hear. I experienced this deeply when I was too ill to eat and stay busy—the emptiness and unfelt childhood emotions I kept at bay with food and busy work started to surface. Oh my, oh my, the bitter sweet surrender in silence and letting go—raw and uncensored.

Unwinding ancestral broken hearts, may allow us access to recreate, re-parent and honour an upgraded version through the visitor called dis-ease. Science tells us change is often uncomfortable until new habits are grooved into the mindbody. When it becomes a new healthy habit, taking it one moment and one day at a time, may help ease the integration until we one day awaken to know, "nothing tastes as good as feeling good feels." My committed hope for you is to glean some valuable information from this book, allowing you to do some deeper exploration towards health, no matter how bleak the prognosis or progress.

Most people who've healed or experienced prolonged remission with ANY disease, often have integrated an internal cleansing protocol, while releasing excess in all its alluring disguises. Many people end up concluding that illness was an absolute gift towards living much more authentically. May this be your story as well.

When we are told illness is a disorder of unknown origin, (idiopathic) and is incurable, all self-empowerment is gone. This is the greatest danger one will ever stumble into! I have pushed beyond this self-limiting diagnosis, as so many others have, and found root causes that I will lay out for you. Most people do not have a clear blueprint of health and are on medication to manage a symptom. Stepping out of "sick-care" management and changing our biology to a higher paradigm is what I hold in my heart for you.

Viewing medicine through the eyes of *Physician Committees for Responsible Medicine*, may catapult us on a new path, as we research food and lifestyle medicine as a safe and compassionate cure, with quick and amazing results![2]

Maybe you feel this cry from deep within your fiery belly, "There must be more!" This is where the integrated learning comes in, witnessed in myself and others for decades: "When the student is ready, the teacher appears." How we honour and partake in life, our breath, and food—from growth to ingestion, is how we do most things. This is my story of love and hope, because friends, once we regain sovereignty, into a new experience of sacred spaciousness, then a healthy and happy EarthGut is possible; imagination and creativeness return, peace is accessible, and we finally realize love is EVERYWHERE. As in the words of Course of Miracles teacher Marianne Williamson, "Our greatest fear is not that we are not good enough. Our greatest fear is that we are powerful beyond measure."

## What Are These Things Called Bowel Disorders and Dis-Ease?

In integrative medicine of all traditions, disease is known to have been caused by toxicity creating inflammation due to some of the following: stagnation, deficiencies, excess, foreign toxic chemicals in our food/environment, etc. which the body sees as foreign and begins to forget its' innate intelligence and attacks itself. The mindbody is very dehydrated and deficient at this point. Understanding and healing this, will make a huge leap in our health and has the potential to give us much inspired hope!!

On the wide spectrum of digestive issues, irritable bowel syndrome (IBS), while not life threatening, can create a life of discomfort and inconvenience. Many people with IBS have normalized an uncomfortable belly, and also have had many digestive challenge points in their lives.

It is estimated 60–70 million people have digestive diseases such as heartburn, acid reflux, gastroesophageal reflux disorder (GERD), IBS, indigestion, constipation, diverticulitis, diarrhea, abdominal pain, etc. To relieve these symptoms people turn to acid inhibitors, pharmaceuticals, and immune suppressants. However, some stomach acid is needed to absorb calcium, digest food, and prevent small-intestine bacterial overgrowth, (SIBO). We need gut integrity. We would be wise to *Listen To Our Gut*, as Jini Patel teaches. Yet how do we relearn this, if we are taught to eternally focus outward our whole lives, instead of to look within?

IBD is categorized by Crohn's disease (CD) and ulcerative colitis, (UC). IBD, at this point in standard medical care, is considered idiopathic, meaning of unknown origin and incurable. It is considered an autoimmune disease caused by dysregulation and hyper-immune response to the host microbiome. Yet when outside chemicals such as glyphosate and internal chemicals created from stress, attack our gut lining, our immunity begins to lose its intelligence.

Ulcerative colitis is limited to the large colon mucosa lining, whereas Crohn's disease can affect the entire gastrointestinal tract, from mouth to anus and move into the concentric musculature of the bowel, creating fistulas and other symptoms such as rectal bleeding, pain, weight loss, and poor bowel control.

**Key Findings from the 2018 Impact of IBD in Canada report (based on Statistics Canada and Global Statistics):**
- 270,000 Canadians are living with IBD and many living with digestive distress.
- By 2030, the number of Canadians with IBD is expected to rise to 400,000 (approximately 1% of the population).
- The prevalence of Crohn's and Colitis in Canadian children has increased more than 50% in the last 10 years.

Canada has the highest rates of IBD in the world. But these are only the ones that seek help, most do not. Many people struggle with their gut and this very personal area gets ignored, shoved down, and numbed with the many distractions and mixed messages of the external world. IBD patients often eventually need surgery to repair damage or remove an obstruction and some end with bowel cancer. Our belly is our intuition, and as "we begin to listen with devotion to its' messages, we become the love which we seek."

Throughout this work, we will explore the systemic disease process that has correlated intestinal mucosa lining inflammation and hyper permeability, (more commonly referred to as 'leaky gut')—as the root causation of the multitude of systemic disease, including illness such as the trigger for autoimmune disorders. Most everyone who is ill has gut issues and are cellularly dehydrated, though many are unaware.

**Our belly is our core connection to the Earth, our tribe/family, and our sense of safety and security, all of which are incredibly unsettled for many. Our base energetic bottoms are searching for belonging whether one is aware of this or not. In the reconnection journey, we may discover a settled sense of what it means to be this spiritual being, having this human connection and that it does matter. We are here right now in these precarious times and we do belong!**

In reclaiming our ease of mind, proper hydration, restoring bowel health, slowing down and showing up authentically, some of these symptoms can begin to be alleviated in just a few days. A bowel and brain at ease is very regenerative in nature.

The way to not "keep being sick" is to stop doing the same thing over and over that created the ill mindbody. In my twelve-step group this is the definition of insanity, to do the same thing over and over and expect different results.

Bowel rest will perform miracles. Changing the inner terrain and reconnecting does also. As Dr. Robert Young says in the pH Miracle: "If your fish was sick, would you treat the fish or change the water?"

**Do we not want to get to the root cause of what is irritating the bowel? It is of little help to us and our healing to believe autoimmune dysregulation just happened to us and we are powerless to overcome it.**

# The Reconnection of Remembering: We are One

We are part of this unified field. We are expressive, diverse, and whole. The modern, medical model has created many specialists and separatist theories that have sometimes created a divided view of how we see ourselves from whole/holy.

Remember the movement WWJD—"what would Jesus do," I don't believe what we are doing mindlessly to the earth and each other. We are being called home to this truth. Jesus said "forgive them for they know not what they do." But first we need to know what we are doing. I believe I can bring some balance and some options that have been deemed miraculous, yet they are simply just natural laws of health. They are here as a reminder of our roles as earth-keepers and the next seven generations unseen or as George Carlin says, "or maybe Mother Earth will just shake us all off like fleas!"

**We DO want to know if the food we are feeding our children and grandchildren is safe and healing! Let us reclaim our mother bear instincts!**

Our healing begins as we connect compassionately to our planet's biome, as the whole interconnected and pulsating network it is. We may begin to ask ourselves:

- **What is my interconnection to Earth? To view the cosmos as a biome, I ask myself, "Is the world I am building, what I want for our grandchildren to inherit?"**

- **Where did the nutrition in our food go? Where are the nutrients in our soil, the spring in our step, the easy smile on our faces?**

Interwoven into this is the understanding that living, uncontaminated, microbial-rich soils are innovators of great souls in motion. We may begin to piece it together that: glyphosate and chemicals in genetically modified organisms (GMO), food, and conventional-sprayed food inflame the entire body and open the tight, single-cell, protective mucosa colon-lining junctions; radiation exposure creates chaos; turning off Wi-fi when not in use and deep breathing helps one feel calmer; and eating and drinking specific substances will affect mood and energy.

We may begin to feel we have personal healing power within the practice of "healthy living" and whole-person reclamation. Whenever the mindbody is disconnected and unwell, we are at a crossroad; to numb out symptoms or "to bring fierce compassionate inquiry and attention upon it," as my favorite "doctor of fierce inquiry," Dr. Gabor Mate, teaches.

Throughout this book we move towards a happy gut. However, since so much of the root of disease begins in the EarthGut manifesting in the mindbody, people searching for answers for their mindbody out of harmony, may find this information of value on their journey as well. People who've connected gut health as the root cause, as the first investigative protocol of whole body healing, find gut health relevant for the treatment of every disease.

When I began to understand how to connect the dots that all the dedicated scientists, seekers, physicians, biologists and farmers set before me, healing began on a whole new playing field and I truly understood:

**When fear sits in the fire of our bellies and bathes in gut inflammation, it makes it incredibly challenging to navigate our way into rest and nutrition. When it is allowed to burn up the rubbish, we will stop burning—deep and kind compassionate inquiry will begin and we are on our way back home.**

May you use these multitude of references and quotes, from just some of the many brilliant and committed physicians and teachers available, because: "When one has eyes to see, and a heart to hear …"

May we begin the vast journey of remembering! Is it found in the gut-brain axis of the Vagus nerve, which affects us mostly from the bottom up? Or is it in the incredible neuron connection and memories of our heart's code, the receptor field of so much of who we are?

May we explore our mindbody with new and deeper reverence. May we know we are loved and accepted. May we reflect this for each other.

Many of our earlier memories are stored deeply within all of our organs, fascia, cells, and microbes. There are mindbody practices to move them through. "Vagal wanderer" is our mediator. Divine self-realization is our mediator. Breath is our gift.

I see in the glazed-over expression of so many people during discussions of our planet in crisis. They are greatly overwhelmed and denial is the coping mechanism that takes over. Yet we are the ones who will be the change, not the politicians or the food safety regulators. My friend Sheryl McCumsey, microbiologist and advocate, has discovered this many times over, when her deep concerns were ignored by people responsible for our health policies and environmental protection. When we get more and more in touch with this and become our own silent observer of our habits, our thought forms, our food growth and our consumption, then we may expand our compassion beyond comprehension and begin to take action. This is not just about haphazardly eating. It is a symbolic representation of how we live our lives.

Imagine how much has changed in our world over the last 33 years. We have developed more disease, dis-ease, and disorders—cancers, IBD, diabetes, depression, anxiety, and sleep disorders—than we have ever witnessed in the devolution/evolution paradox of human-unkind/human-kind. Brain disorders such as dementia and autism are at an all-time high, rates of diabetes are rapidly increasing, all leading to our health care and basic productivity on a path to destruction! Is there a link within our missing microbes?

Consider how our living ecology is suffering: more contaminants than ever are present on the planet; a disconnection of thought from our "heartland" and agriculture into conventional dead-lands to feed our ill animals. We have lost more than 55% of our earth's living diversity in just the last 50 years, one species extinct every 20 minutes! This catastrophe is reciprocally reflecting in our lack of microbiome diversity and failing health. What we do from here on matters! We can affect the changes we so desperately need for our children and all life forms on the planet; from our EarthGut restored intelligence! From this crisis, opportunity and microbial mystery will graciously lead us home.

# *The Invitation: Bacteria Intelligence*

You are invited on a journey, far beyond the realms of white-knuckle willpower, failed diets, and inflammation. This exploratory healing, chlorophyll-rich "green-land" has the potential to heal our EarthGut, cravings, emotional disharmony and dis-ease.

When our inner ecosystem—our microbial terrain, is thriving with good bacteria, we can achieve balance, we feel good, love and joy are returned, and we have the potential to heal our affinity towards drama and over consumption. We may choose to meditate instead of medicate with overeating, stimulants, and distracted behaviour. This allows us to find the quiet place within, where microbial remembering begins, for

**we cannot accomplish peace in a sterile, disconnected environment.**
This primordial divine truth resonates into our living nature farm soil,
while building our microbial inner garden. In every moment we are faced
with a choice: to strengthen our connection or wither.

There are many books written on healthy eating, yet why can only a
few of us adhere to the principles? This is a question worthy of attention.
As it turns out, many of the answers have been found in our microbiome.
This is also the new paradigm shift of understanding our oneness through
microbes, shifting the understanding of mitochondria into the lens of our
trillions of bacteria and how these bacteria cross talk. Through resonance
and cohesion, we have landed into a world so desperately in need of
microbial communication, re-establishment of healthy flora and fauna, and
ancient microbial healing. It is here addictions thrive or dissipate back into
the nothing.

**What if the root of cravings and lack of communication at a cellular
level begins within our missing microbial diversity and loss of gut
integrity? What if the loneliness and loss of connection we are forever
feeling, began within our missing biome?**

If we become curious listeners—enough to bear witness to healthy
microbiome habits—while breathing deeply and lovingly into them,
we may find an entry into this glorious world of commensal bacteria,
abundant energy, health, and calm. As a reciprocal force, communication
throughout humankind may be restored.

"Eat dirt and live" may be an adage for life as a positive connotation,
in the days so near, as we feast from local home and peace gardens. Pure,
peace-farmed vegetables resonate with the frequencies of prosperity and
give us the ability to thrive. It is now known a healthy gut can thrive with
70-80% or more friendly bacteria, leaving invaders helpless, as shared in

the brilliant book, *10% Human: How Your Body's Microbes Hold the Key to Health and Happiness.*

We are now left with a choice, to research and explore truth or accept the status quo of ills and pills. In rebuilding our gut's thin single-cell protective mucous membranes, we have the opportunity to begin where Hippocrates suggests: "All healing begins in the gut. A wise man should consider that health is the greatest of human blessings, and learn how, by his own thought, to derive benefit from his illness."

Disease rates are rising so very fast, and as addictive as denial is, this can no longer be excluded. If we are to reclaim our sovereignty, happiness, and health, peace, love and microbes offer us a well-lit path through the dense fog of contradictory advice.

# *We Are One:*
# *Understanding the Microbiome Unity*

Understanding the microbiome is the beginning of deep reverence for our infinite healing powers, and it is only with hope restored that one has the motivation towards self- empowerment.

The human gastrointestinal tract (GIT), known as the microbiome, is lined and protected by 100 trillion microorganisms or more, which hold structural integrity; assist in metabolic functions; and intestinal mucosa immunity, to name just a few.

In the beginning were microbes, ever-changing, diverse, life-giving. It has been said that Adam was created from the dust of the earth-microbes. We are over 90% bacteria with a multitude of bacterial gene expression, which depend on the environment they are exposed to. We are dust in the wind, earth, recycled light.

The microbiome, as revealed in much research, has been shown to be able to modulate mood. Our bacteria are needed for the breakdown and utilization of nutrients from breast milk onward.

Individually, we are composed of 20,000 genes, yet one gene, depending on its environment, can make 200 variations of protein. On the other hand, our global worldwide diversity has two million gene expressions as well as 40,000 species of bacteria, 300,000 species of parasites with 1.5 million gene expressions, and 5 million specified fungi with 125 trillion genes and the granddaddy—ten million times more viruses than there are stars![1]

How do we fit into this complex web of DNA information? We can take comfort in knowing that, in the words of Dr. Zach Bush, "If they were out to get us, we would have been gone a long time ago!"[1]

The microbiome role in health and disease has been ground-breaking and vastly researched as a "forgotten satellite organ" of paramount interest; yielding perspectives yet to be fully understood: in the modulation of all disease, endocrine function, and gut-brain connection. The human microbiome is fundamental in what humans are to become; diverse and thriving or inflamed and frustrated.

As we explore the role and mechanisms in which the microbiome and beneficial bacteria function, how can we not feel awe for the work it is performing for us! In our microbiome alive, we are currently degrading from toxins, educating ourselves on immunity, modulating all mindbody functions, and satelliting our organs into systemic/metabolic health.

Worthy of further exploration is how our cultural amnesia perceives real food. But empowering mindbody practices and knowing **microbes as our friends** has some of us searching for more effective solutions through our EarthGut interconnection. [3]

- Microbes ferment undigested fibre/carbohydrates, synthesize vitamins, and neutralize toxins, while producing key small-chain fatty acids (SCFA) which respond as food for colorectal tissue, assisting in maintaining tissue integrity.[4]

- Gut bacteria has been linked to the ability to influence mood, modulate neurotransmitters such as GABA, and control the SCFA histamine, a main generator of serotonin/dopamine, two mood enhancers primarily produced in the gut).

- The microbiome has the ability to synthesize SCFA from the plant fibre prebiotics we consume, (assisting insulin, glucose, carbohydrates) such as acetate or butyrate, and propionate.[5]

In pondering, we may ask:

- **Can a prebiotic (fibre) and probiotic (for life) rich diet, and the reduction of pathogenic bacteria and pesticides, along with reduced stressful thought and inflammation, promote a healthy microbiome and, ultimately, disease disappearance, and be the precursor to our deeper connection?**

- **If we heal the integrity of the gut, will we heal the integrity of humankind? Will we become more human-kind?**

- **May we alter our stress responses and happiness level by feeding the joy-inducing microbes?**

Viewed through the lens of the microbiome, disease appears to have a systemic link into one's individual diet and nutrition, exposure to antibiotics and pathogens, stress, surgery, microbiota early development, and a lost connection both to this microbial-rich earth as well as each other.

Many of our earlier memories are stored deeply within our organs, cells, and bacteria, as gene expressions through microbial interface. There are trillions of gene expression of bacteria, viruses, and fungus, within our global diversity. We are forever connected through microbes and if every virus that comes along flattens us, we may want to have a life makeover. Each and every choice we make (or environmental factor that bombards us), formulates the next generation, leading us either closer to a health collapse or toward awakening.

These microbes may change quickly via food, thought, stress, chemical exposure and sleep. They react to our environment such as chlorinated chemicals and medication in water, SAD (Standard American diets), loss, loneliness, processed food, electromagnetic force (EMF) and chemical/pesticide stress—thriving on the opposite.

When we listen to our gut instincts, while frolicking in the grass and swimming in electron-rich waters, we are freeing our children from nature deprivation and we are back on the right track, possibly the fast track. This ancient microbial unwinding gives us much hope! We cannot possibly be separate or alone on this one beautiful blue ball hurtling through space! Yet many of us feel alone. If we do not have healthy connections, we will make unhealthy bonds with addictions and pathogenic bacteria. We will lose our gut and heart integrity.

# *"Change Is Good, Donkey"*
## *~Shrek*

## *(Well, Not All Change)*

I truly believe change is happening quickly and we are coming home, with a longing to live in a healthy world where our children can be well, happy, hydrated and free from the over-stimulating world of deception and chemical food substitutes. I believe many of us, despite this chaos, are hungry for change. Parents are tired of junk food vending machines in school and food companies adding addictive chemicals targeting our children. I believe parents will soon be teaching their children to love being in the trees over the screens. We are illuminating the hidden sugar and addictive negative stuff, for it is not empty calories but rather negative calories, for the body must use much life force, brain health and nutrition to detoxify them. I have faith we are hungry to reconnect in the healthiest way yet, maintaining the integrity of our bowel, our breath, our brother and sisterhood, our biome!

Changing our diet is hard, but illness is much harder. Support may be the key to shifting! By embarking on a seven-day juice or water cleanse, while silencing, resting, meditating, we may be resetting our telomeres and fears! When we change, our biology can also change very quickly. We can change thoughts with interruptions of a constant mantra and affirmation, when fear rears it dark cloak: "Every day I am stronger, I am at ease and free! I am enough!" We change in meditation just simply by not running from ourselves anymore.

The paradox is that the more sovereign we are, the more we realize our interconnection. When we get support, we feel stronger. As social-designed humans, unplugging emotionally from social food can be really tough.

I know this very intimately.

The journey may be incredibly bumpy, for chaos will always be a huge part of change, and an essential one at that. The other greatest obstacle for myself was living within a world that often supports the disintegration of health and promotes addiction. Eventually we learn to have food, fresh green juice or smoothie, and something to share, with us on our journey throughout the day.

Addiction is a symptom of disconnection, and the food industry has paid huge money to formulate addictive, processed edibles. Big pharma benefits from our not knowing this. Yet there are healthy communities awaiting.

We are biochemical individuals. One can feel amazing on fresh green juice while another will have flaring diarrhea. Instead, this is an invitation to explore how peace, love and healing our microbial world, into an awakened living, can have a profound ripple effect.

Microbes and molecules are our shared unity, connecting us across the universe and resonating through every breath we breathe, every smile we share, every garden we grow in peace for all, and in the words of Whole Earth Catalogue Editor Stewart Brand: "If you don't like bacteria, you are on the wrong planet."

We are microbial earthlings, billions of us—70 trillion cells rich, with enough potential to completely liberate our birthrite for peaceful connection—successfully arresting inflammation and disease of many names and faces. My deepest desire for you is to be well. I believe our highly intuitive and nerve-rich belly and bowels are getting our attention fast! Will we change what is not working?

**The war on bacteria is over**. A new revolution is taking place in every corner of the world, calling us back to a sweet remembrance of microbial-rich, plant-strong medicine and soil. This is our beautiful ever-changing body electric! Let's take care of it so we do not age in a sickly state. Let us cultivate living land together.

## *Maybe Health Was Just Not Taught*

I wish for you, the reader, to have an understanding of the link between all human disease and a dis-eased, restless, disconnected world and poisoned conventional soil. May you see autoimmunity dysregulation in a new, brighter, and more hopeful light. These three adventurous musketeers—peace, love, and microbes—have been well understood by many as the remembering journey towards healing. It may seem like a far-fetched thought that these alone can regulate inflammation, yet research throughout this book, our understanding that disease is stress-related and much documented study, within integrative medicine/meditation has made the connection unquestionably clear.

You may be reading this book because you have a bowel disorder that you are unable to keep in remission, or have chronic systemic inflammation. May this book leave you with a fierce compassion to connect to new possibilities to help heal yourself. Disease begins in the EarthGut mindbody, even when we are unaware of this.

Specialists are not wrong: they just lack sufficient nutrition and mindbody education. I love my gastroenterologist. She is kind, brilliant and really does care! I was very sick and she believed I would never be well if I went off medication. I am suggesting a balanced, multidimensional healing protocol designed to heal root causation. I am writing this for her too and all the physicians who care, yet were not taught this information; and for all patients whom she says may not have the motivation to make the changes I have.

By no means is this medical advice. I may have needed prednisone, biologics, or 5-aminosalicylic medication when I was very ill. Medication can be a bridge as it has for me, illness a messenger—to change a life into one that is authentically ours. Having made the journey to renewed health myself, and quick recovery when I go off track, I am just returning to pay it forward. In humble grace, may I offer other ways that do not further damage the microbiome as many pharmaceuticals do over time. This is the decade of microbiome research. This is the decade of reconnection. You are a trailblazer.

I have repeatedly experienced the skepticism from allopathic doctors when they ask what medication I am on for Crohn's. When I explain I keep it in remission through diet, mindbody lifestyle, meditation and prayer, I am frequently met with irritation when I say these have healed me; as if I was saying something so bizarre, so risky! Yet fast forward 12 years and the last MRI revealed thickening in my rectum was gone and an absence of scar tissue. A miracle? Yes, an awakening miracle—a rewiring miracle. This book is a call to release the past and begin a new way of navigating life. I am not the first. We are many.

We may be left wondering why we were not told beforehand, in the medical circles, the way to empowerment and wellness. Please allow that question to fuel you with a new passion for study that you may have never felt before, leading you to the how of healing as it did for me. Enormous amounts of the how are available to you and really do work.

**The key that unlocks the world of infinite healing is this … our deep participation is a must in this journey! Within this process, the victim must leave and the old and debilitating question "why me?" must be replaced by "show me."**

This is the game-changer, my friends. I promise! Enjoy the journey, for she is calling us home! Come, beautiful soul! It is the microbial reconnection you are looking for. Come home to our beautiful and ever-forgiving Mother Gaia. Come home to your heart. Truth awaits there. Have hope, reach out, minister each other, have faith, and do your part.

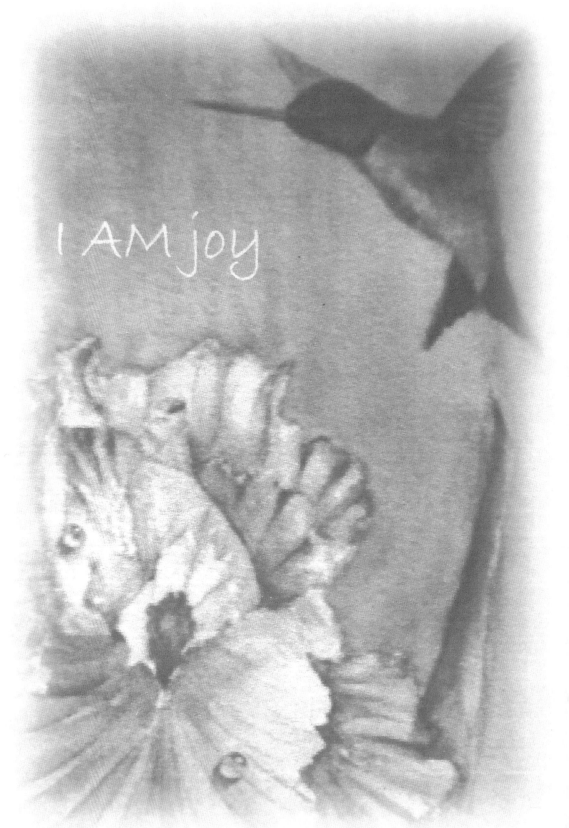

I AM joy

*The Story of Peace, Love & Microbes*

# How this Book Reads:

## *Affirmations, Meditations, Questions, Stories & Science*

Some say we are what we eat. But, as I am constantly reminded that we are what we believe, think and value. These determine not only what we eat but, to a large degree, how our life will unfold. Have you ever noticed what you reach for when you are stressed and how that changes when you feel at peace?

We are not just a collection of molecules, we are also light and energy, and everything our mindbody does requires us to have a high-density mineral field, sufficient hydration, and the quorum of beneficial microbes for our body's energy to shine into health. In the light of this understanding, this reading is intended to offer many thoughtful questions and quotes to ponder as a call to action.

In the passages throughout, meditations and gratitude affirmations are suggested as a game-changer for many people. In these visualization meditations, bringing all senses into the process, including the feeling sense, is of essence towards remembering your healed state. To end each meditation visualizing two or three people that would benefit also from you being well, and imagining the positive impact on their life from you being healthy, is the groundbreaking work of Jose Silva and the *Silva Method.*

You may record your voice as you speak these affirmation meditations and go barefoot onto the earth and listen. Notice how the sound of your voice changes as you heal deeper. The truth is, most of us are telling ourselves something all the time; therefore, why not talk to ourselves in relaxing, healing and loving words? The "I AM" words can begin to reprogram, as we reclaim our goodness, which was always there. When we move into deeper states of meditation, we may experience the transcendence of the "I." Yet while we're continuing with our self-talk, let it be gentle, a much kinder and softer inner dialogue. Invoke what you want out loud. Reprogram the self. "I am healing more every day!" Then let your biology come to life! My two-year-old grandson does this so intuitively! When he wants his brain to really absorb something, he repeats out loud, until it is remembered; such as the arrival of his new sister as she lay in a pillow in his arms he repeated dozens of times, "Mommy, if Phoenix gentle with baby, Mommy be happy?" Months later, he remembers gentleness. I see it click into his brain even when he is feeling rambunctious.

I experience this truth of body self-talk and the body's reaction to our inner dialogue when I direct massage therapy clients to their breath and their body begins to relax, muscles soften. This changes quickly when they begin to think again and suddenly much to their unawareness, their neck, jaw, and shoulders start to tighten again. When they become aware, people find it quite interesting how unconscious tension is connected to harsh inner dialogue, creating their body's stress. Then, right smack dab in the middle of all this is an accessible place, a place beyond our prosecutorial mind, that arrives on the next gentle, mindful breath.

In David Hawkins' *Power vs. Force*, understanding the power of moving from apathy and fear to integrity and appreciation, we begin to experience that what we focus on, we create. Visualization is known to be just as effective as breath-work and meditation in working with IBD. Neuroscientist Dr. Joe Dispenza is one of my teachers of this truth, bringing the abstract image into manifestation. Can you visualize yourself calm and well? Can you envision what you are like in this healed and empowered state? Will you let go of "Why me?" and shift to "Show me!"

Ahhhh, the stories shared. Stories are amazing teaching and healing parables that often have a cathartic effect (I am not alone and there is hope), especially in a world continuing to claim that there is NO CURE. We all love stories. Stories can connect cultures and teach us ways that respect dignity. May your stories be ones of healing and letting go of the rest, the history that we lug around. For it is known that reciting negative events puts large amounts of stress hormones into the mindbody.

Then, alas, there is the poet! Poetry and prose has been a way for us to both listen and hear deeper into our heart. Writing inspired prose has always been a lifeline for me. It is a way to convey from one heart to another heart. May the prose of this book find a way to your heart, your poetic remembrance!

Then, there are the questions! Questions we may have for that answers give us a clear directive. Then there are others we may never be able to fully answer. Yet when we live quietly, or are hungry for change, within the question we may be open to deeper and deeper truth. Remember to ask the question that Futurist Barbara Hubbard pondered after being given a glimpse of future humanity in 1966, "How may we use all this new power for Good?"

May you find blessings within this deep understanding of "as above, so below," moving beyond our story into holding out our hand to walk another home. Within the space between words, may we expand the power of gratitude.

Suggested homework includes ways to turn intention into verbs. For there is one thing I have come to know: **we cannot hold onto stress and paralysis at the same moment we are living in gratitude and conscious change**. Even in times of extreme illness, we still have our beating hearts and breath to be grateful for, and simple nutritional choices to improve our health, such as fresh green juice. I focused on just those two things to get me through my crisis, with much relief.

In these writings, old marketing norms are extinct, and sacred commerce and interconnection prevail. I choose to bring experts together here to honour and promote united souls within the abundance of their quotes, research, healing protocols and stories of hope. A colleague who read this manuscript said, "Whose book is this? You speak of so many others and why should someone read your book over Robynne Chutkan?" Dr. Dispenza would say: "I believe we are all geniuses." Within sacred commerce, we all stand united in the opportunity to turn our lives all around.

This book is also sectioned into four parts: peace, love, microbes and healing protocols. Please feel inspired to read as you wish. Compel yourself to further explore other doctors and researchers who have moved beyond conventional pharmacology study into integrative medicine health. We are all in this together, just walking each other home. **Rewrite your story**.

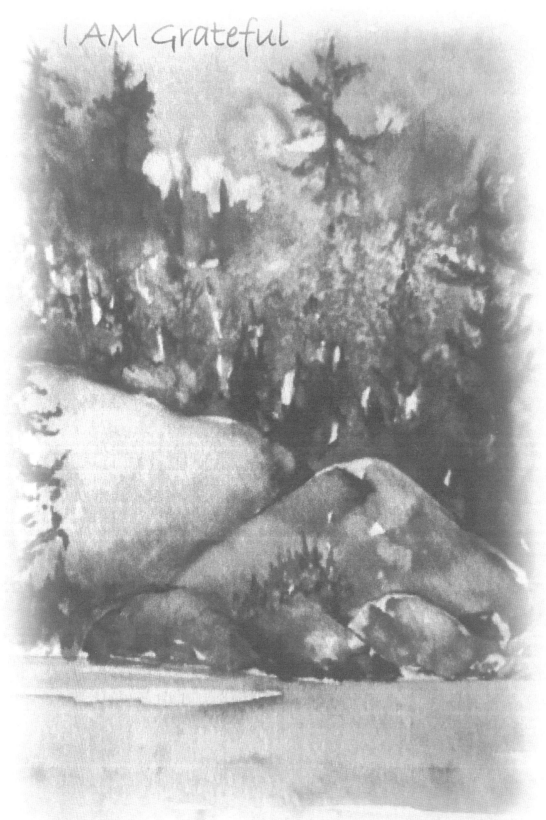

I AM Grateful

*Preface*

*by John Phillips:*

## *The Cosmos as Biome*

What if we look at the universe as an extension of the living world within us and around us? What if the universe is nothing but a greater expression of the life we know as human beings? Suppose we are but a micro-scale of the macro-expression that forms the universe? Does the adage "as above, so below" become an inquiry that leads us to examine
the world as an expression of all that is within and without us? In short, what if the cosmos and the biome are one?

One law of the universe seems to be "Life begets life." One paradox of that Universal Law seems to be the observation that as stars form and planets evolve, life seems to evolve from inanimate matter under favourable circumstances; at least, as far as we know in the instance of our own planet. In *Holism and Evolution*, the thesis of a holistic pattern of evolution is given when Jan C. Smuts observes that "… from inanimate matter, life evolves, and from simple life forms, conscious human life has emerged." Smuts noted there seems to be an intrinsic pattern built into the process of evolution that works to create greater and greater wholes. Human beings are but one example of this tendency to create ever-better-organized entities that express ever-higher levels of organization and consciousness. This tendency in nature and the universe to evolve ever-greater levels of organization, function and consciousness was defined by Smuts as "Holism," and a superior force in evolution compared to the Darwinian view coined by Herbert Spencer, "survival of the fittest."

The cosmos then, seen from the point of view of holism, is evolution's manifestation of the greatest whole and the greatest consciousness. The paradox of life evolving from inanimate matter resolves by understanding that the term "inanimate" is an illusion. Consciousness is universal and intrinsic to all things in the cosmos. *There is no such thing as life. There is no such thing as death. There is no such thing as inanimate matter. There are only transformations of form and shifts in consciousness.* Consciousness is the unified field of all existence, all non-existence. Even empty space, the void, is full of consciousness. It is our limited perspective and awareness that constrains our understanding and experience of the innate, intrinsic, all-pervading existence of consciousness.

Human beings, as a microcosm of the cosmos, appear to have the ability to evolve a consciousness that reflects the cosmic consciousness of the whole universe. There are many terms used to describe this phenomenon, such as "Enlightenment" and even "God Consciousness." But the best way to describe this experience may be "Awakened Being," the state of existing in an awakened consciousness that is aware of being one with the universe.

Awakened Being is not an otherworldly state of altered consciousness, but the peaceful acceptance of the truth; that the true nature of human nature is the realization that living a conscious human life is but a minute experience of the conscious life of the universe. Such a life has its cycles, its rhythms, its beginnings, its endings, and its renewals. Like the spiral dance of the planets around their stars, like the whirling dance of galaxies and dervishes, Awakened Beings experience the whole and the part as one. All time, space and being are but the cosmic dance of the one cosmic dancer.

As an Awakened Being, when we examine our human existence, we note first the existence of our bodies, even as the infant is fascinated by its fingers and toes. We become aware of others outside of ourselves, and gradually we become aware of the world around us. This world is teeming with other beings, other life. Some of it is intrinsically evident or visible and helps to form the world as we know it, with all the features we need to survive. Air to breathe, water to drink, food to eat, shelter, and other needs that are met by the external world in which we exist.

There also exists an invisible world equally important to our survival as human beings: a world of organs, microbes, cells, and atoms that is hidden in plain sight as an integral part of our human existence. Invisible forces are also at work: gravity, nuclear magnetic resonances, wave and particle reactions, subtle organizing energy fields forming patterns and organizing atoms and particles into greater and greater wholes. There is also the invisible world of thoughts and emotions, expressions of invisible bodies and realms of existence that gives us knowledge and feelings about the world inside and around us. Within our bodies, there exists the microbiome, a consortium of living things that dwells inside us, in our guts and even in our bloodstream and organs.

The origin of this biome is the life that surrounds us. As an infant, we are inoculated and colonized by a variety of microbes: from our mothers, from the air, soil, food and water we take into our bodies, and from touching the world around us. This biome is vital to our existence, helping us to digest our food, helping our bodies ward off diseases, and performing many other life-enhancing functions that affect even our mental and emotional well-being.

We barely understand the vital role of the biome within and around us. We hardly comprehend that it is vital to our existence and our survival. Yet, as a species, we are presently doing many things that threaten to destroy the very biome that keeps us alive and healthy. We need to awaken to the fact that our continued existence and future evolution depend on understanding, preserving, and sustaining the biome. Human beings are not separated from the environment, nor are we separate from the biome surrounding us. As the environment around us sickens, weakens, and eventually collapses, so do we.

The illnesses that plague us and destroy our health and happiness only reflect what is going on in the world around us. If we are going to heal ourselves, we must heal our relationship with Gaia, the earth mother who brought us into existence. *We cannot be healthy and whole in a world that is being destroyed in the name of making profits, where the highest value is greed.*

Dr. Gabriel Cousens, MD, ND, has inspired the world with his teachings of *Conscious Eating, Sevenfold Peace*, and the Six Foundations as the basis for creating a "culture of life," the counterpoint to the *"culture of death"* status quo driven by a value system of materialism and the egregious accumulation of wealth at the expense of the biosphere. In our current Anthropocene era, this culture of death is resulting in an astounding species extinction event unprecedented in earth's natural history. Never has one species by its actions and impact on the biosphere resulted in the extinction of so many other species in the biome. Eventually, as more and more species go extinct and ecological functions die, the human species itself is impacted, and our survival becomes questionable. We have blindly cocooned ourselves in our material world, and are perilously failing to recognize the fact that *the most endangered species on the planet is very quickly becoming ourselves!*

In his book *Sevenfold Peace*, Dr. Cousens points out that the first peace we must embrace is "Peace with the Diet." The food we eat is key to our survival, health and happiness, not only on the level of the physical body, but also on the level of our mental/emotional well-being; and even on the level of our existence as multidimensional spiritual beings. Reviving the food culture of the ancient Essene tradition, Dr. Cousens has promoted the use of authentic live foods in the form of sprouts, ferments, nuts, seeds, vegetables and low-glycemic fruits as the basis of a raw vegan diet to promote health, happiness and longevity. Rudolf Steiner warned us in his lectures *On Agriculture*, that the adulterated food of the future would make it difficult for humans to think properly and to act forcefully enough to stop the damage to the environment that would jeopardize our own existence. Pioneers of the organic gardening movement, such as J. I. Rodale and Robert Rodale in America, and leaders of the Nature Farming/Natural Agriculture movement in Japan, such as Mokichi Okada and Masanobu Fukuoka, helped to initiate new paradigms in food production that return to agriculture's holistic roots. Dr. Teruo Higa of Okinawa, Japan has helped create an Earth-Saving Revolution using the benefits of effective microorganisms (EM), a mixed-culture probiotic microbial solution, as a core technology for creating and renewing "living soil." Indeed, it is the basis for a regenerative organic agriculture that returns farm soils to the pristine status in the climax ecosystems found in nature in the forests, mountains and prairies. EM is used also to create probiotics for human health as well as serving as a tool for environmental remediation.

As a student of Dr. Cousens' School of Holistic Wellness, Tami Hay has written a masterful work sharing her personal healing journey and her discoveries in her book *EarthGut: Story of Peace, Love, and Microbes*. Tami Hay shows us that all healing begins in the gut, in the microbiome within us that reflects the biome around us. *EarthGut: Story of Peace, Love, and Microbes* can help many people who suffer from digestive disorders gain the insights they need to help themselves and others. It is a work filled with love and inspiration and concludes with a very helpful appendix containing recipes and practical tips on how to succeed with a live-food diet. Enjoy the journey reading this fascinating and inspiring book, *EarthGut: Story of Peace, Love, and Microbes*. In peace!

John Phillips *Gardening for Peace* www.gardeningforpeace.com

The seeker relinquishes seeking,

sinking deep into the

ancient resting place of a blessed heart,

many lifetimes, around and around,

yet knowing it now,

as if for the first time.

~ *Tami*

*The moment one definitely commits oneself,*

*and then providence moves too.*

*All sorts of things occur to help one*

*that would not otherwise have occurred.*

*A whole stream of events, issuing from*

*the decision of rising in one's favor all*

*manner of unforeseen incidents*

*and meetings and material assistance*

*which no man would have dreamed*

*would come his way*

**~ W.H. Murray**

# To Begin:

# Making the Commitment to Wellness & Epigenetic Cures

## Commitment to Self-Healing and Toxic Reduction

We cannot speak to the commitment of unplugging from food, habit, substance … unless we address the resistance and the saboteur that rears its wild head whenever we choose to move into a deeper level of conscious living. A wise mentor Cyndi Dodick once said, "Maybe one day someone will do a thesis on backlash." She laughed and added, "I call it front-lash now. I can see it coming."

The saboteur has many names: resistance, the shadow, procrastination, self-sabotage … yet we have infinite healing power to change and rewire.

We are energy and light, with infinite access to shift our biology quite quickly. Commensal microbes are our remembrance, our allies. Resparking the light of our mitochondria—the biology of life—is our remembrance. Love is our remembrance. Mindful awareness and chewing thoroughly is of essence. All of which, when fed and strengthened, shift our biology into health, despite what we are up against.

You may feel this rebel "resistance" creeping into your mindbody at the thought of change, especially the unsettling topic of letting go of eating and living patterns. I have never felt so much resistance in people, as this topic evokes: primal fear patterns of lack, starvation, going without! To the contrary, we are strengthening and healing! If we give food less power, one little loving sigh at a time, we find strength we never knew we had.

Change is hard, but illness and disconnect are harder yet! We come up against resistance every day. Let us explore how to move right on through while continuing to meditate on compassionate living and loving ways of life. This is the road less travelled, yet now well sought out.

The microbiome is here to assist in this detoxification and is a vast contributor in honouring and supporting the body's amazing self-cleansing and self-healing systems. We increase the electrical charge of the mitochondrial energy through fasting, movement, meditation and re-hydrating. In being the silent observer of old habits falling away, we find strength to go on.

Our body is an incredible self-healing organism! If our autoimmunity is on overdrive and attacking itself, what are the invaders? If knowledge empowers us, then we must free ourselves from medical models of symptomatically treating diseases. What we do not eliminate we recirculate. When we do not seek knowledge, we may slide into the vortex of unnatural immune responses.

Toxemia, in natural hygiene, is suspected to be caused by some of the following: incredible lack of self-knowledge and self care, dehydration, our agricultural killing fields, (18.9 billion pounds of the water-soluble glyphosate alone is sprayed and leaking into water and air), broken hearts, overeating, over vaccinating, a polluted world, toxic EMF overload, insufficient internal cleansing, and lack of rest.

When given a break, the bodies can self-heal miraculously. I have observed this time and time again, in myself and many others. Self-healing happens best in nature, quietude, resting, and supportive rejuvenation centres and community. Sometimes this is messy and emotional, yet what we can feel, we can heal.

Here on this planet right now, we are exposed to substantial amounts of toxins that have deep and very dense roots in the gut. Our lack of connection has us going to the dry wells over and over, and usually at the expense of our planet. Some of the medicine is here. Drink it in, bathe in it and smile once again. Commitment is a verb and requires health habits of self-love.

## Epigenetics & Inflammation

We are all unique people with individual biochemistry, whether it be genetic hereditary traits or epigenetic programming. But how we interact with our environment is the most important factor in understanding how our moment-to-moment choices affect our wellness. This is the pioneer work in the new field called Epigenetics currently being studied by developmental biologist Dr. Bruce Lipton. Epigenetics (meaning over the genes) has revealed that more than 90 percent of our health is dependent on how we interact with our environment.

The epigenetic blueprint is the protein that surrounds our cells and interacts with the environment. One cell may have as many as 200 protein expressions, depending on its environment. This allows us the opportunity to understand the importance of taking responsibility for our health instead of feeling disempowered by our genetic blueprints. This is also witnessed in the life-saving discovery of micro RNA, how microbes are communicating and adapting to the infinite dumping of toxins in our environment in an attempt to save us. Once thought of as "junk DNA," which do not make a gene, these turned out to be helpers: 15% of the micro RNA in blood vessels are from bacteria, 15% from fungus and 5% from food modulating, cross-talking with bacteria. God does not make junk!

There are many committed scientists feeding us microbiome research. Some of this groundbreaking research is the work of a physician whom I study, and deeply trust, Dr. Zach Bush, and M Clinic, research lab and satellite teachings.[6] He is working within the paradigm of understanding the microbiome role in hydration, nutrition and connection—reiterating the critical role in re-inoculation through visiting as many diverse ecosystems as possible.

The world is in a state of big change and chaos. **We learn through observation. As children we are in theta, hypnotic state until approximately seven years of age. We learn through watching and doing what others around us are doing. Therefore, we must be gentle with ourselves as we reprogram. We must use the power of grace and stay connected with like-minded souls who are wayshowers of liberation.**

Inflammatory habits may easily turn into addictions—we often crave what we are over sensitive to. Many diseases are diseases of chronic inflammation and disregard the natural laws of hygiene and nature. Inflammation is our body's response to invasion and we do not have to look very far to see the integrity of all our immune defences are being invaded. Allergens and food sensitivities, if unchecked, can result in constant chronic inflammation, systemic integrity breakdown.
Peace, love, and microbes may be the antidote for a world of now.

I AM
Grateful

"There is no path to peace.
Peace is the path."

~ Gandhi

# Chapter 1:

## *Peace*
## *Culture of Life &*
## *Sevenfold Peace*

*When the longing for peace becomes greater than the desire*
*for distractions, we are on our way back home.*

## *Why Are We Talking About Peace?*
## *Three Key Learnings on Peace:*

- Peace is the antidote to stress and since most health issues have deep roots in stress, taking three nice focused breathes when feeling overwhelmed, and choosing calming food and drink, is a game changer.

- Peace and quieting enough to listen, has the potential to impact everything in a reciprocal relationship with our microbiome, our world, and every cellular interaction within all systems.

- Starting every action with an intention to have a peaceful respectful outcome, creates calm; for we are all in this together.

## 11 Peace Builders

1.  Just deep breathing consciously is enough;
    meditation / silence / listening / reconnection

2.  Heal intestinal hyper-permeability (leaky gut) to feel peace

3.  Let go and let GOD (good orderly direction) this requires trust
    in the process of a world awakening and a loving Universe

4.  See beauty everywhere

5.  Respect sovereignty

6.  Make peace with food, family, and the moment
    (organic / veganic / plant based )

7.  Keep gratitude going (in mantras, in journals, and in
    every interaction)

8.  See the spark of Divine in everyone

9.  Collect your microbiome diversity in the peace of nature and in
    food growth and preparation

10. Live peace through reconnecting

11. Choose peace over any other goal

# Exploring an Amazing Model for Peace:

# The Essene Sevenfold Peace:

How do we create peace by being peace, as Rabbi Cousens speaks in his book of the same title? We set up our lives in a way that allow us to touch that still place within. We breathe, drink, eat, think and act in a way that helps us remember something beyond overstimulation. **This is the time to live and speak truth!**

*"Blessed is the child of light
who is strong in body,
for he shall have Oneness
with the Earth …*

*He who hath found peace with the
body, hath built a holy temple*

*Wherein may dwell forever,
the spirit of God"*

~ *The Essene Gospel of Truth*

What we do to the planet, animals and atmosphere is a direct connection to what we are doing to ourselves and each other as author Dr. Will Tuttle so clearly shares in *The World Peace Diet*.

I truly understand the magnitude of the task at hand. To deepen our individual peace practices, in a world such as ours, may change everything. One thing we do know for certain: the way we are going about our lives is unsustainable, for our personal health as well as the planet. The Essenes knew this peace as a sevenfold practice. This is true of all traditional medicine, such as the balance of the four directions of the Native medicine wheel, Ayurveda medicine, and traditional chinese medicine (TCM). TCM is a 3,000-year-old practice of medicine, in which the immune system is known as "Wei Qi," flowing in the tissue, back and forth, from the lungs and skin to the intestines.

The Essenes, a group of spiritually grounded people dating back to the 2nd century B.C., supported conscious community, and lived within the natural laws of hygiene and sustainability. They understood that health includes the aspects of individual peace as Sevenfold: peace with body, mind, family, community culture, ecology, loving Creator and earthly mother—all within global peace and harmony.

Many people on their health journey feel alone, especially if they are too ill to want contact, stuck in a hospital receiving no nutrition or too weak to make real food. As I write this, two sacred souls in my town, sharing *The Green Moustache Restaurant*, are bringing real organic, plant-based food into hospitals!

A safe warm haven and a circle of support are critical in the wellness journey. The sevenfold peace practices are essential in times like these.

Many of us have never been taught the foundations for well-being. Many highly educated people have a complete disconnect from how their body works, or the most healing nutrition, or even what breathing for wellness feels like. Most have no clue what is in our water, air, food supply, minds. But wanting to get well or to avoid more illness, many begin to understand that modern medicine could only bring them so far.

Feeding our body and minds in a way that enriches and maintains a healthy microbiome will give us a much calmer perspective on life. Choosing peace and love (beginning with the self) may allow us to move away from the 'herd mentality' (everyone else is doing it, so it can't be that bad for me), and begin to question the chaos.

Peace is inclusive and "once we know, we can no longer pretend we do not know." May these writings encourage you to embark on a healing journey through a whole-food, plant-based diet, along with peaceful practices that promote a healthy microbiome, allowing us to receive love and hope—full circle. May we each find our way to the peace and truth that cultivates a healthy microbiome journey of liberation.

## 🍵 Food for Thought:

If everyone in the world ate plant-based meals once a week, there would be enough food to feed the world. There is enough food to feed the world when we are not using it to feed farm animals. The greatest contribution to greenhouse gas emissions is the methane in cattle flatulence, not emissions from vehicles. We have enough food! Farmers are being paid to not grow food! Is eating so many animals and drinking dairy a hoarding of resources? We are one compassionate choice away from healing our EarthGut. What will we each choose next?

# *The Culture of Life*

In the present state of our global environmental health and food crisis, the calling to reorganize ourselves in a way that aligns with a wellness path is about coming home to our pure child-heart that existed before judgement, neglect, addiction and resistance! We will enter this freedom as children, healed and open-hearted.

The peaceful warrior's job is to alleviate suffering, darkness, and despair. The culture of life is one of deep communion, opening the floodgates to spiritual forces, connecting our physical temples to our divine dharma, our true life-purpose. The sevenfold peace is a spiritual discipline that can be created and cultivated by each individual who chooses to be peace.

The personal has always been the political; while peace, deeper peace, has always been an inclusive endeavor—from choosing to eat foods from organic, microbial-rich soil to refusing to participate in a world that supports violence. This means creating our own quiet, trained and non-violent bodies and minds as our gift to our beloveds: our children, our communities, our global brothers and sisters, loving Creator, earthly mother, and the next seven generations unseen. For how we do one thing is how we do everything. Steeped in communion, we have the opportunity to cultivate a world of "eternal presence"—beyond our small self-identification.

**I once read of a jovial monk who escaped exile in Tibet. He witnessed the murder of most of his monastery and birth family. When an interviewer asked him how he could be so joyful when he witnessed so much terror, he answered: "because it feels good." The path to creating peace by being peace feels good!**

Many of us have been raised, during our deepest theta, hypnotic years, in the other communities, the ones that are sleepwalking. It is a leap of faith and an act of courage to separate from the distractions of that world and heal old childhood programming.

It is in childhood we learn to connect or disconnect from ourselves and the sensations of our mindbody messages. Feelings may have been too painful to feel when we were little people and had minimal power in our lives. Knowing this can allow us to develop the practices that support "fierce compassionate inquiry."

Essenes believe in cleansing and seeing wholeness. Abraham Maslow believed someone became a whole person when they ONLY saw someone's pure potential. Shamans know they can only hold space by helping a person remember their healed state. Pure focus has the power of the flowing springs of life.

I was raised in the forest in a small community in northern Ontario Canada. When I wasn't studying frogs or trees, I was swimming in a nearby river or fresh, cold spring lake. The daily cold plunges, like those practised by the Essenes, felt like a baptism, and still do to this day. I have adopted the "Finnish Way" of cold plunges each morning as a deep calming practice.

I learned later, eating mostly vegetables and eating lightly would be of great value in my bodywork and the art of healing. I have been weaving my dharma into bodywork, for the past two decades. My clients can always sense my 'vibe' or how grounded I am. Eating lightly allows the light to come in.

The ancient Indigenous ways may be the undercurrent of much of the healing art practised to this day. I feel this when I gather hot stones for massage. As we become more sensitive, we feel the strength and teachings of the ancients, all has life and everything is part of us. Traditional plant medicine and elemental healing was and still is a significant part of most traditional indigenous cultures throughout all time.

**Each generation is given the medicine out of crisis. Plants are our medicine, love is our epigenetic glue.**

# *Peace with the Body*

Anyone awakening into healing knows health is a mindbody connection; the mindbody-belly-heart-spirit interacting continually. Making peace with our diet is our gift to our body. Dr. Gabriel Cousens shares that it usually takes about two years before the physical body establishes peace and stability with vegan high-vibration live food. Dr. Zach Bush confirms this in his struggles and later triumph in going plant based. A peaceful process and reconnecting with beneficial bacterial diversity, makes the transition easier. Peace with our diet is the point, and possibly our primary way out of our global crisis. This is a challenging job, to begin such a massive life transition of values. Finding peace and keeping ourselves calm will really help.

*To keep the body in good health is a duty, otherwise we shall not be able to keep our minds strong and clear.*

*~ The Dalai Lama*

I am still here, making peace every day. For some, food may be the greatest addictive obstacle to overcome. For others, living below the poverty line and in food deserts, real food may be impossible to buy. This is where we take our body back to the soil as our fore-mothers did and reclaim our rights to grow our nourishment; sprouts, nutrition-dense vegetables and other foods. In a nearby city Edmonton, a dedicated man began the architecture and teaching of edible yards, replacing grass often treated with chemicals to kill some of our greatest medicine, including dandelions.

Thoughts of changing what we eat is a heated subject! It triggers people! Refocusing changes emotion quickly from where it is trapped as "mind-grasping."

I like to embrace "grasping addictive patterns" as I do my little sacred two year-old grandson; to refocus him gently saying, "this instead," making the "instead" fun and joyful.

Abstaining from food indefinitely is not a choice, as abstaining from drugs are in drug recovery. Research done and shared throughout this book does indicate a green juice or water and fast for short intervals, such as five to seven days, can reset all unhealthy eating patterns, allowing addictions and our mucosa colon lining to heal much quicker. Yet, it is our day-to-day mindful choices that decide whether we will change our food cravings and habits. Food companies know this and create fake food that biochemically ignites addictive brain responses. It is important to understand this when wanting to heal the root cause of addiction. Avoiding substances such as sugar, unhealthy fat, alcohol and salt that set up the mind-trappings and chemical cravings very quickly, would be a wise choice. Not keeping them in our homes and thus avoiding them in our loving mealtime preparations, is key. An acidic, dehydrated body creates cravings that may have us craving sugary junk food for a couple of weeks after just one or two days of imbalanced emotional eating.

*"In making peace with the body during this transition, is making peace with the mind. From the perspective of the Sevenfold Path of Peace, a harmonious process is more important than how quickly the goal is reached."*

*~ Rabbi Gabriel Cousens*

# *Conscious Eating: Peace with the Diet*

It would be deceiving to write about nutrition alone, for nutrition is the symbiotic conductor in this orchestra. My exploration has led me in the direction towards understanding the power of building a great friendship within the silent quietude; daily enjoyable movement with conscious breath; sweet resonance of music; love-centred community living, and a healthy microbial-diverse bowel. This may reconnect us to the divine heart, Mother Earth and her diverse ecosystem … our awakened truth.

Conscious eating is about curiously exploring our diet and developing the right action for a very intimate lifetime relationship with food and its planetary impacts. For food becomes our biology and changes our biochemistry in such a way that we either become energetic and purposeful, or tired, irritable, dehydrated and acidic: marked with highs and lows of cellular neurotransmitter depletion. This biochemical change happens quickly! We can literally begin to change our biology in 24 hours for better or for worse by eating super-foods or by an unhealthy food and stress binge!

When daily habits are ones of addictive overstimulation, we are no longer free. We are trapped, externally focused and easily controlled. Right thinking, alkaline bodies, and reduction of inflammation give us back our freedom to choose a calm, connected harvest haven; a remembering, if you will.

Choosing a non-harming lifestyle allows us to shine light into a world in desperate need of illumination, for it is difficult to feel sick, dehydrated and inspired in spirit at the same time. Food is our soon-to-be biology, our quiet friend or foe. It either sets us free or traps us. What we think, drink, eat and do has the power to build our bones, blood, brain, breath and planet. It is a circular cause-and-effect action.

While knowledge is everywhere, knowledge regarding diet is vastly contradictory. It is like a huge smog of choices that sometimes lead us into a scattered state of paralysis. Some diets promote high, good fats while others support a low fat, higher carbohydrate. The one diet that has outlived all the fad paleo and high or low carb diets is the science and spiritual ancient/modern knowledge of whole-food, plant-based diet for the healing of all diseases.

Most people find the information on GMO/GE food and pesticide used to be too vast and controversial to explore and fall into complacency. We are in a health crisis that we can never financially, spiritually or physically support. We must vote with compassionate choices. Knowledge with action can translate into health.

One thing remains clear—no diets for health promote processed white sugar, white flour and food additives. Kindness requires that we omit foods that result in harm. Denial is illusive. Questioning can create change:

- **How does restoring the gut mucosa barrier change our level of joy and hope?**

- **How does eating from the light, healthy microbial-rich biodynamic menu and being hydrated make you feel?**

- **How does walking barefoot in the grass, deep breathing in the microbial ecosystem, culturing food or working living, rich soil feel inside our bodies?**

- **How does swimming in an electron-giving fresh lake or stream awaken energy? I always feel much calmer and much more alive!**

- **How does being free and clear to love deeply change everything?**

Our conventional food source is contaminated with health-destroying chemicals and pesticides, therefore moving towards real organic/veganic food while supporting regenerative soil practices, is the healing salve mother earth is needing as we restore nutrient-rich living topsoil, lost in North American conventional practices. Starting with a small garden pot or jar of sprouts is the beginning!

Extensive research has concluded that the best diet in the healing of any disease is a plant-based, enzyme-rich, hydrating, nutrient-rich food, as used in the leading healing centres around the world. Many fad diets have come and gone or have been revised with new names. The oldest and most extensively researched authentic diet that heals is a plant-based, whole-food, highly enzymatic and mineralized diet of Earth-based sun-food.

A reconnection diet includes diet of the mind: meditation, emotional clearing, and finding ways to feel connection and in-joy-in-my-self. Therefore, right knowledge is about living and integrating universal truth, listening to our EarthGut instincts, honouring detoxification as the first line of defence to heal disease and beginning to understand what my new friend, Barry learned when wanting to be medication-free and heal after a heart attack, we must be ready to do the work ourselves.

Especially for women in today's culture, making peace with our diets, hence our minds, is a much-needed act of love for humanity. This can help move the feminine consciousness from pseudo-materialism and narcissistic beauty into a deeper feminine purity of purpose. Understanding our bodies as complex, living organism that need clean fuel, deep restorative sleep, and connection; allows respectful understanding as we move in the right direction.

I am one of many who have sustained a respectable remission with IBD through a vegetarian lifestyle of predominantly live food, herbal cultivation and enzymatic, mineralized food. I am building energy, or prana; with such practices of deep belly breath and energy cultivation, spiritual guidance within community, and silence through prayer, yoga, and meditation, while supporting others to do the same. I sway at times of crisis, but return. I have a well-lit path home. May we all light the way for each other.

## Global Body

All food and drink that brings that keeps our energy unblocked is both a local and global act of love, and requires much ancestral unwinding from "desire and craving." Releasing instant gratification for long-term peace is the way, yet it can feel mighty challenging at times!

*"The body is an ecological unit, as a planetary cell in our global organism and the cosmic body."*

*~ Dr. Gabriel Cousens*

The mindbody is studied within the universal principle, "as above, so below," and is considered to have a global connection. The mindbody healers use rest, pure food, water sources that deeply hydrate the mindbody, exercise of conscious movement, sunlight and earth energy, and access to fresh air. All of these are accelerated through breath work and must not be undervalued. Our loving, calm reconnection may be the alchemist recipe for a life rich and balanced in emotional, mental, and physical health, and divine purpose.

When we are at peace with our bodies, we have found a diet that promotes ahimsa, (non-harm) and peace with our EarthGut. We now choose infused cuisine, rich in both pre and probiotic plant fibre and microbial builders. We know that by keeping our gut flora strong and diverse, we are living a type of freedom that many people knew well before the introduction of conventional-processed and genetically modified food.

We learn that by feeding the good bacteria, we are starving the ones that have the potential to harm us when out of balance. The array of prebiotic flora-building healing plants and herbs are held in high regard. Eating this way is the most significant choice we can make towards global peace, the health of our earth and ourselves.

*"There is seemingly only one choice,*

*the choice you make."*

**Rameen Peyrow**

# QUIET HEART

*Listen my child, be quiet and still*
*Has the sun risen and gone without you feeling the warmth of me?*
*Not a moment with a quiet heart?*


*What if it has never mattered what you do?*
*But how you do it*
*What if life meant no longer sleep walking and idle talking?*
*And everything you do leaves you closer to yourself,*
*every other, and Earth Mother*


*Awaken to this work at hand*
*Feeling the mystery in the bigger plan*
*For when the doing and the do-er meld*
*We know for certain we are held*
*Because, my child*
*There are no ordinary moments*

# Peace with the Mind

## Mind Training

*"Mind not, my child, the noise of this world.*
*For it changes like this gentle breeze or storms astray.*
*For surrender delivers it all on the wings of a dove… a place of unarmored,*
*uncensored love."*

*~Tami*

All teachings emphasize mastery over our thoughts as the most significant part of our evolution. The thoughts we send out resonate throughout the cosmos and we are responsible for whether we want to entertain these thoughts. Meditation has the potential to release us from mental slavery and has the ability to siphon thoughts and no longer accept inferior ones. Meditation is our healing balm to soothe our ulcerated wounds.

"Energy follows thought" is the reminder often shared with my clients, as they bring their attention to the tight spots and imagine them softening. We also chuckle at how their body tenses every time they begin thinking. Possibly for the first time, they become aware of how thinking often does not support peace of mind. Thus begins the inner work

*To become more authentic, practice feeling the difference between true heart connection and surface level connection with others. When you feel anxiety, go to the soft place in your heart. Breathe in feelings of calmness for a few minutes. Practice sharing your love and care without expectations. If you fade on your intentions, go to your heart and reboot your commitments. Breathe in kindness, care and compassion to raise your vibration throughout the day.*

*~ Heart Math Institute*

from mind trapping to mind training.

Our hearts and minds are linked directly to the field, the matrix of the planetary mind. When we really let this truth settle deep within our hearts, our breath, our blood and our bowels, then we truly understand how much of a planetary impact we have by keeping our minds clean and connected to loving-kindness, and we take responsibility for our energy. As in the brilliant book, *My Stroke of Insight*, Neurologist Jill explains how having a stroke in her left brain, heightened her intuition. In the months of preverbal recovery, she was able to feel deeply the hospital caretakers who gave her love and energy and those, who through their shutdown hearts, took energy from her. This changed her path into one of which her mission is to teach the importance of what energy we are bringing to the world!

It may be impossible to control our thoughts until we purify our body with organic nutrition! My dear friend Kim told me after following a pure diet for three months to heal Crohn's, her mind became peaceful, and her constant mind-chatter began to leave.

If we begin every interaction and every daily transaction with a quick three-breath invocation of imagery of peaceful words received in love, we may become the change we wish to see in this world. This practice not only settles the heart and mind, but also relaxes the nerve firing in the gut. We then begin to obtain a quiet mind and heart. We stop idle talking and walking, and understand that everything matters. We begin the remembrance walk home. Sound simple? Not so much, yet much simpler than always dealing with

*Feelings can be placed into two categories: those that create energy and those that exhaust it. The feelings that create the greatest energy are love. Manifested in terrestrial nature, it gives all that is necessary for health. The Essenes considered the thinking body as man's highest gift from the creator.*

*~ Dr. Szekely*

emotional residue from reactive states of inflammation.

## *Peace with the Family*

To love another unconditionally is our greatest task and our greatest accomplishment, for conscious and sacred union into what will heal the planet. When our family is one of harmony we can rest. Ancient medicine is steeped in this truth.

Our resonant energy field creates peace or chaos. Families are our training centre to develop mature love, resiliency, commitment, shadow illumination, and we can support as individuals in reaching spiritual mastery. Conscious coupling and parenting are the greatest gifts we can give the planet. As Jesus spoke … "When two or more get together in my name and pray." The power can be 100-fold.

Yet, I must admit, many families were more like "survival of the fittest"! I know this intimately. My children, grandchildren, and spiritual family has been my place of nourishment now. We all can join in health-minded community now and support each other, teaching nutrition, ministering and renewing. Being a loving conduit and steward of mother earth and each other through keeping our hearts broken open, while encouraging people alike to do the same, we learn about our feeling bodies and our interconnectedness to all life.

*Let thy love be as the sun
which shines on all
creatures of the earth,
and does not favor one blade
of grass for another.
And this love shall flow as a
fountain from brother
to brother…
He who hath found peace
with his brothers
Hath entered the
kingdom of love.*

*~ Essene Gospel of Peace 2*

We are social creatures, with a deep longing for belonging and love. For many this may mean building communities to support, witness and counsel our journey of a thousand miles. When we obtain this, we become healthy members of a humane community and we heal our past.

*I build my childhood space*
*Resilient Child I AM*
*Space-boundaries and pain ignored*

*Ahhh– yet space found ME*
*Outdoors—up a tree*
*Bacteria Alive*
*Under expansive skies and butterflies*
*Earth my reprieve*
*Time and space, the respected illusions they are*
*HERE*
*I can feel ME*
*Amongst the logs and polliwogs, the violets and buttercups*
*The rays, the moon*
*Hours of Oneness*

*Here I weave God's wonderlust!*
*All sparkly and full!*
*Here you found me ... All sweet and free*
*Here we melded into ONE*
*Weaving and weaving*
*God's wanderlust love*

Families are the people who share our lives, community and hearts. The highest level of relationship evolution is intimacy. The root of "intimate" means "to know" and all beings thrive when they are truly seen. To say "I see you" and really see the other, is what is the deepest experience in intimacy, as in a favourite scene from the movie Avatar.

Many years ago when my daughter was four and we were dropping her nine-year-old brother off at hockey, he said—what felt like out of the blue, "Why do Pete and Michelle never argue?" They were our closest family friends. I was a bit dumbfounded yet before I could respond, four year-old Jennifer piped up, "That is because they know each other!" To see and experience intimacy within ourselves and others, we must see deeply within our hearts, and see "the other" through the child-heart.

Family love can achieve enduring, accountable, peacemaking relationships and awakened purposeful love. It is the commitment to work through the "other stuff" that allows the family to stay, play, and pray together. Family allows us to do our mirror work, build more solid foundations and grow where we are planted. Yet first we must be accepted! Some of us are unable to do this work in our biological families, which has often been a causative factor in disease and much suffering. If we are to evolve and to make peace with this, we will find our spiritual families, and on a soul level, will mutually support our spiritual awakening and evolution.

# Peace with the Community

*With all your pearls of love*
*And much heartbreak healed*
*Dark turned to golden threads of love's sweet whispers*

*Go forth my child, into the world*
*And let your heart-light shine*
*Onto the weary and forlorn*
*The lonely and forgotten*

*Let your healed scars*
*Bring sacrament to all children*
*Illuminated and seen.*

People are awakening everywhere. Community gardens are "sprouting up." Organic/biodynamic food is found everywhere—this is awakened love. As we align our consciousness during this planetary tipping point, our thoughts of kindness and service allow our souls to receive the messages of global healing, which includes the treatment of every sentient being. This is inclusive of the animal world. If we knew how to have complete health on a holistic diet within a thriving microbiome, then would we be able to give up our addiction to animal eating? This transition may take up to two years to develop the microbiome diversity to support plant-based nutrition, yet the journey can be rewarding beyond measure!

We receive in order to give. There is a universal truth as *Quantum Physics* author Gregg Braden says, "We are compassionate by design and if we come upon the uncompassionate heart, we must understand the wounding that must have been endured in order to have forgotten."

Braden reminds us in his book *The God Code* that each of us has our own unique God code which only we can bring forth through the infinite power of grace. Peace with culture is an intuitive and sometimes very vulnerable process.

Let us see God-given gifts in each other. Let's help each other become the healthiest and wisest people we can cultivate. The investment into "becoming wisdom" is in pure food, water, and loving action. Sowing seeds of love will allow us cultural rebirth.

The children we are raising today will determine our destiny. It would be wise to ask ourselves if fast food, violent media/gaming and degrading competition will achieve our goal of becoming the healthiest and wisest we can be? Will these choices draw us closer? Can we create our family gatherings of rainbow nutrition, nature, laughter, and love?

## *Peace with the Culture*

The Essenes, indigenous peoples and mystics had pathways into the awakening culture. They heightened their intuition through studies of the mystics, prophets and teachers, nature and plant medicine, art and literature masterpieces. They honoured all directions of wisdom and knowledge, while paying homage to the sacred and divine in all life.

*Stay together friends. Don't scatter and sleep! Our friendship is made of being awake.*

*~ Rumi*

We are living in a world of cultural forgetting as referred to as the "culture of death." This may sound extreme, yet the number of seriously ill people is climbing rapidly and this truth is impossible to overlook. Ulcerated colons and cancer are showing up more and more in babies. This is a tragedy.

If we awaken to this deeply suppressed truth, within an understanding of our woven interconnection, the rivers of truth will wash away all the tsunamis of betrayal and seeds of deception. She awaits so patiently our return. When we participate in circles of chanting, drumming, singing, cultural ceremony, eating pure whole food, then that awakening evaporates race and cultural differences, and dismantles war and illness. Transcending separation is befriending healthy ego. Without separation, oneness prevails. This is very threatening to a herd mentality, yet it is happening despite the chaos we now see.

The rampant anxiety found in our culture has a direct correlation to the anxiety and suffering of the animals we are inhumanely raising and consuming. Peace is difficult to cultivate and very costly to achieve in this distorted and anxiety-laden energy exchange involving the consumption of feedlot, caged, and mutilated animals. Awareness of truth is essential.

# Peace with Earth Mother—the Ecology

## RETURNING

A movement is erupting
As we go deeper and deeper still
Gaia responds, earthworms return
Humble farming, authentic nature farming
Wellsprings of wisdom rising

And we bow
Back through the microbial twines of truth
Truth-tellers speaking from each direction
Of minimal tillage, diversity and microbial-rich Mother Earth

A microbiome wellspring—Un-poisoned
Our forgotten organ remembered, Restored
Humble hands and hearts—joining

Going deeper and deeper still

Diverse webs, biosynthesized peace practices
Kuan Yin speaks of compassion for ALL
Gardens of Peace
GARDENS OF PEACE

Nurturing clean, accountable practices such as organic/regenerative lifestyle, renewable resources, and peace practice matters. If it requires 660 gallons of water and ten pounds of grain to make one pound of meat, we must rethink our eating practices and consider the

*The earth is not just the environment. The earth is us. Everything depends on us knowing this or not.*

*~ Thich Nhat Hanh*

words of Eckhart Tolle: "We either become enlightened or extinct."

70 billion animals are imprisoned and slaughtered inhumanely annually, nearly 10x the human population and as the reciprocal circle, are creating imprisonment of human disease. Perhaps our greatest addiction is what Osho has identified: denial. Will we allow the truth to set us free, restore peace?

## Questions

- Can we act consciously and compassionately on behalf of our children, from whom we have borrowed the earth, right here and now?

- Can we speak for ecological life-giving and sustainability, which the Ancients knew many moons ago?

- When we make a commitment within ourselves to maintain peace wherever possible as our main goal, do we accept innovative, intuitive ways to respond and guide us?

- Will we allow ourselves to feel this intuition, deep in our belly, directing us to whether we are listening or not?

As we return to being the students of systems, nature, and gardening—we shift into a global community of earth keepers. We move into living a life of harmony within the natural forces. We shift into internal and external peace in our world. There is a biome diversity destruction theory that connects lost planetary diversity and the missing beneficial

*Man is governed by the laws and forces of nature. His health, vitality, and well-being depends upon his degree of harmony with the Earthly forces.*

*~ Szekely*

microbes in our gut. This connection is worth meditating on.

**We may also find it inspiring to reflect on the Hopi Prophecy, written as a prophecy teaching for this time. It has become a creed for my life:**

*You have been telling people that this is the Eleventh Hour, now you must go back and tell the people that this is the Hour. And there are things to be considered...*
*Where are you living?*
*What are you doing?*
*What are your relationships?*
*Are you in right relation?*
*Where is your water?*
*Know your garden.*
*It is time to speak your truth.*
*Create your community.*
*Be good to each other.*
*And do not look outside yourself for your leader.*
*Then he clasped his hands together, smiled, and said, This could be a good time!*
*There is a river flowing now very fast.*
*It is so great and swift that there are those who will be afraid.*
*They will try to hold on to the shore.*
*They will feel they are being torn apart and will suffer greatly.*
*Know the river has its destination.*
*The elders say we must let go of the shore, push off into the middle of the river, keep our eyes open, and our heads above the water.*
*See who is in there with you and celebrate.*
*At this time in history, we are to take nothing personally, least of all ourselves.*
*For the moment that we do, our spiritual growth and journey come to a halt.*
*The time of the lone wolf is over... Gather.*

# Peace with the Loving Creator

I have yet to meet a person who has found their way through chaos and dis-ease that has not called out, surrendered or given themselves over to something greater than their own will. To know the higher self is an integration of the material, feeling and thinking body, into oneness. The universe with keep putting up roadblocks if we move away from authentic flow.

We may have felt this great oneness in cold water electron cleanses, suckling babes, childbirth, rebirth, dream time and body entwinement with beloved, preparing food lovingly, feeling a sense of belonging and purpose and loving and being loved… many blessings. Yet others feel completely alone in their journey. Illness with all its messiness and unpredictable bowel stuff can be very isolating. Yet even a couple of days of a healthy elemental diet, bowel rest or light juicing can reduce the spastic bowel considerably.

A sacred personal journey is meant to bring us peace. If this is not the case, it may be wise to find a benevolent loving Creator in these times. GOD—Good Orderly Direction—a place to rest, a place for inspired action, a place to be our best, dissolve, reform and dissolve again.

*May GOD self-realization be the final aim that all humankind will one day achieve.*

*May we all be inspired to listen deeply and take right action, by implementing peace throughout our lives.*

*May we compassionately and gently shake that massive tree of dis-ease out by its roots, replanting ourselves in rich, mineralized microbial soil.*

*May we all be part of the change; connect through prayers, meditation, and right action.*

*May we find a peace so deep and so wide, we hold space in our hallelujah heart, to call many home, heed the Hopi prayer and gather ourselves, live in sacredness, truth, peace, and love. And so it is.*

**Story by epigenetics Dr. Bruce Lipton when working his way through college in a garage:**

"The problem is this—when we go to rid ourselves of symptoms, we are pulling the light out. The symptoms of your body are your body telling you that you're under stress; that's clear, but the point about it is your body is trying to tell you the symptom is stress and inflammation.

Almost five o'clock, everybody wants to go home and this woman came in and she'd been in a couple of times before. This is her third trip for this issue, a little light on her dashboard says 'service engine' and she got very upset by this and started to go through all the stuff. One mechanic brave guy says, 'I can fix it,' so he takes the car to the back bay. He gets inside the car, he goes under the dashboard and he pulls out the little light bulb and then he has a smoke and hangs out. After about 30 minutes he brings the car back out front and says it's fixed and the woman got in the car and guess what, she was happier than anything! She drove away and the damn light didn't come on again, yet the problem is this—when we go to rid ourselves of symptoms we are pulling the light out -the symptom is just the information that something is going wrong. If you cut off that information about the symptom you're telling the body, **I'm not listening to you! Think what's the body going to do!**"

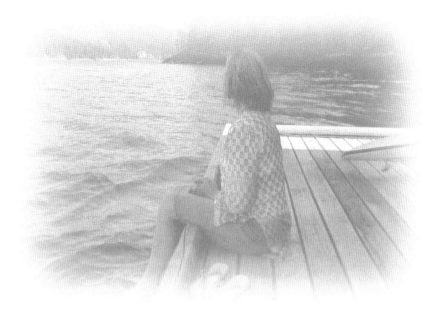

## Meditation:

Closing your eyes, sitting on Mother Earth we realize ourselves as the interconnected synthesis of both Heaven and Earth.

We allow ourselves to feel the three-part breath of belly-to-heart-to-brain, breathing in expansion, and breathing out release.

Every breath in, feeling space and expansion.

Every breath out, a letting go.

In this stillness we experience how just a few minutes of bringing awareness, expansion and release into our body settles our brain, and therefore our infinity receptors to stress.

And we whisper, 'may all beings be filled with infinite peace, may my conscious breath refill vessels of light everywhere.'

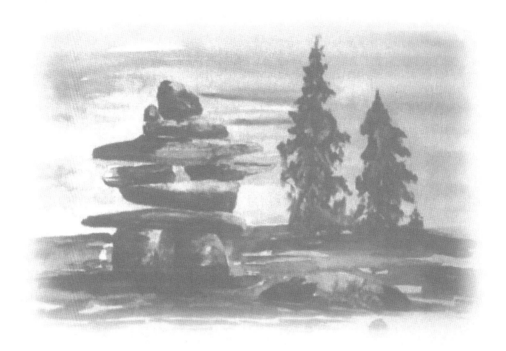

## Gratitude:

I AM grateful for the ability of clear thinking, a Divine presence and the return of peace in times of challenge.

I AM grateful for the infinite peace I can access over and over though breathe.

I AM grateful for the peace with all my relations.

I AM grateful for the act of eating for peace.

I AM grateful for the peace that comes from bringing awareness to my breath alone.

I AM healing and growing stronger every day!

I AM....

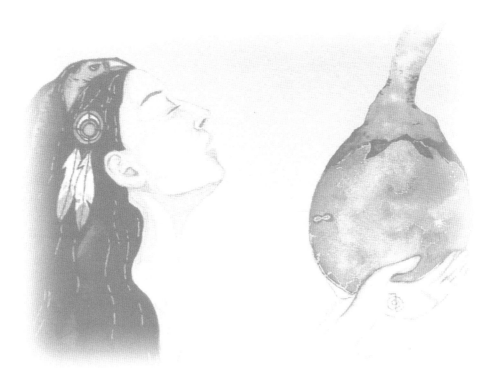

## Coming Homework:

Today will you get your RPM on—rise, pee and move/meditate, just 3-33 minutes first thing, rehydrate with lots of pure water and electrolytes.

Today will you visualize a health thriving you and journal a healthful purposeful day; knowing what you can imagine you can create? A morning practice and clear direction creates healthy possibilities.

Will you prepare your rainbow organic food with daily gratitude, being prepared with food on hand when hunger comes, "lead me not into temptation"?

In mindfulness, one is not only
restful and happy, but alert and awake.
Meditation is not evasion; it is a serene
encounter with reality. Feelings come and go,
like clouds in a windy sky.
Conscious breathing is my anchor.
It only takes three mindful
breaths to come home

~ Thich Nhat Hanh

## Chapter 2:

# *Using Breath-work, Meditation & Integrative Lifestyle to Release Stress & Digestive Distress*

## *The Meditative Breath*

The following is from meditation yogi Sattva teacher Rameen Peyrow, offering his wisdom and elegance of the language into breathing:

"The language that my breathing speaks is an opportunity because, as we know, our breath is actually a part of our human mechanics; it's a part of who we are from now and forever. To begin, we recognize the wealth of knowledge that exists within the breath, void of the decision-making mind and how the rhythms of the breathing can teach the mind clarity. Within that simple act of inhale and exhale, we begin

*I believe we can breathe in the magic of our worth and I believe we can exhale anything we feel we didn't deserve.*

*~ Xavier Rudd*

to self-soothe, and self-soothing is an incredible leap forward within your personal development. It enables you to stay in connection… in communication… with this authentic experience of who you are. The self in this right-now moment, this development, this ability to become very present within this moment and then applied to your meditation practices, elation and interest builds!

It does do that in its own way, different from thought, from emotion, from body comfort and relaxation. It is interesting on its own… and the development of the ability to connect to the elation of conscious breath enables you to see this present moment with your eyes closed or open— void of any other input.

Knowing that you will probably have a thought—and you may even have feelings as you're meditating, but what becomes the hub or the centre of the meditative moment—which is occurring, is actually framed by your breathing; which gives an incredible amount of insight to the self-inquiry component of our meditative experience.

Within self-inquiry, we want to develop the ability to observe, and the ability to observe is enabled through the action of letting go.

We must enable the action of letting go, so that then the breath can assist in the moving through of thought, because the breathing is that of a subtle energy. And when I say energy, I mean something which is moving. So, in that function of your breathing, you are constantly in a state of movement, just like the river: inhale, exhale, inhale, exhale. A thought comes in, a thought goes out, a thought comes in, a thought goes out… and we allow ourselves to go into a trance-like state, just like as you would sitting on the banks of a river and watching the ripples of the water go by.

Often we attempt to see just one ripple as it goes by and then we fix our focus so we can see the entire body of water moving. And we want our breathing to teach us how to do that within our meditation.

Watch the body of water, which exists within the mind, move an energy which is flowing… continuously flowing… and within that dynamic action it produces stillness from the deepest perspective. Your breathing rhythm soothes anxiety and worry. Your breathing allows fear and trauma a place to move out and through the deep breath—just relax or refocus.

Bring full deep breaths into the body, while keeping the eyes closed. Bring your gaze into the space just there in front of your eyes and then use your breathing to enable the ability to maintain this integrity and focus for just one minute."

Meditation is the epigenetic glue that binds mindbody integrity. Mindfulness practice has been used by ancient cultures for thousands of years, as a way to move beyond stress of the sensory 3D reality. Much of this is done through some form of meditation and breath-work, whether it be accessing higher realms through combining breath work and yoga, chanting, drumming, rattling, dancing or stillness. The nervous system can reset itself every 20 minutes, the body heals in a parasympathetic state, meditative breath soothes the mindbody. The meridian energies reset every 28 minutes and the breath can re-regulate itself with only a few deep breaths. The vagus nerve, as we will explore in later chapters, is deeply calmed and tonified with breathing practice and deep breathing awareness. This is the art of remembering, clearing our mind, resetting our nervous system and understanding that by changing the microbiome towards "pro life," an illuminated truth flows into places previously unknown.

I have become familiar with a breath-work practice transcendental re-birthing, (TR). Hosting groups of TR practitioners has allowed me the gift of witnessing people having access to much of their unknown subconscious, releasing trauma through deep and focused breath.

# The Mindful Gut

There have been more studies connecting mindfulness to reduce stress than one may recite. One study from the North Carolina School of Medicine looked at seventy-five women with IBD and put half on a mindfulness-based program and the other half in a support group with a half-day retreat on IBD. After eight weeks, the mindfulness group's symptoms dropped 26.4%, compared to the 6.2% drop in the talk therapy group. The reduction in symptoms in the mindfulness group lasted over three months. Does stress reduction change the taxa of microbes? It has been known, in much research, to change the composition of the microbiome relatively quickly.[7]

*"This God energy is the ultimate food, and meditation is the ultimate digestive process. Meditation aligns and expands the subtle bodies, allowing the cosmic prana to come into our chakras with little resistance."*

*~ Dr. Cousens*

Dr. Braden Kuo, a gastrointestinal researcher at Massachusetts General Hospital, incorporated mindbody yoga, breath-work, and meditation in a nine-week study of IBS/IBD—nineteen patients with IBS and twenty-nine patients with IBD. The astounding results showed that 1000 genetic markers that are associated with IBD were shifted towards reduction in inflammation, with less genetic margins for IBS. This is significant research connecting the power of mindfulness to not just change epigenetic blueprints, but actual genetic markers. It leaves one in awe that the genetic composition, through lifestyle, along with stress reduction, put out the fire in our intelligent and intuitive gut.[8]

An abstract in 2017 on *"The Effects of Stress and Meditation on the Immune System, Human Microbiota, and Epigenetics"* concluded the following results after a two-year study with a variety of people and database:

Psychological stress typically triggers a fight-or-flight response, prompting corticotropin-releasing hormone and catecholamine production in various parts of the body, which ultimately disturbs the microbiota. In the absence of stress, a healthy microbiota produces short-chain fatty acids that exert anti-inflammatory and anti-tumour effects. During stress, an altered gut microbial population affects the regulation of neurotransmitters mediated by the microbiome and gut barrier function. Meditation helps regulate the stress response, thereby suppressing chronic inflammation states and maintaining a healthy gut-barrier function.[9]

Often stress, fear, loneliness and procrastination set us up to "emotionally eat," which adds to physical digestive issues. Therefore, meditation and unplugging allows us to eat in a way that feels quiet and aligned. We are not just emotionally eating food, we are emotionally eating our way through life, and this causes life to eat back. The antidote to this is bringing our awareness back to our breath, food and conscious eating while journaling daily. Within every breath is a miracle-minded opportunity, even a minute of deep breathing will start to reset the nervous system and begin to ignite the "relaxation response."

I have yet to meet or study with a teacher who has not discovered that meditation is the key to dissolving the denser energies that stop the flow of cosmic energy from entering our system and clearing our dis-ease. Meditation has been the main way for many practitioners to build prana and release codependency.

When everything one studies and practices in regard to healing and wellness, (in this book and others), connects stress reduction and quiet mind, as the venues most important to health, it may be wise to touch into our breath regularly and let go, even for a few seconds. If we were raised in stress or work in stress, making the longest journey from our head to our heart/body and simply just focusing on our deep belly breath in and out for even a minute, throughout the day, is a game-changer.

When done in a conscious meditative manner, breath significantly increases life force, whether it be in gardening, preparing food, loving our children, and loving ourselves enough to just let go for even a bit. Bringing awareness to deep breathing is our vehicle.

## Yogic Breath-Work, & Posturing Our Life: No Longer Feeling Like an Imposture:

Meditation and yoga are a life raft to wellness, detoxification of mindbody, and calming of the spirit. The word yoga is derived from the Sanskrit word "'yog," meaning union or oneness. For many, the yogic practice is a method of self-inquiry which may help one self correct much more easily.

*The vagal nerve is deeply stimulated, tonified and calmed through yoga and belly-deep breathing. This is very essential for our wellness.*

### Asanas

The Asanas are one of eight limbs of classical yoga. Asana are yoga postures that assist the yogi in deepening awareness of body, mind and surrounding environment. The spine is known in many traditions as the river of light and energy. These stretching postures increase the flexibility of the spine, but also strengthen bones, stimulate immunity and circulation hence freeing fascia lines (such as in the Yin yoga practices). Asana postures open up the energy channels and chakras.

This increases the opportunity to hear our body's intuitive message and, for some of us, to begin to reconnect with the body awareness we may have lost when society began telling us how to think, feel, act, and behave. For many of us, this did not allow us to hold on to our innate child knowing. I am also aware—through years of massage therapy—that people will only stretch as much as they allow themselves to feel. Memory is stored in our fascia and is much better out than locked in.

Asanas are performed with breath, and are conscious builders if done with concentration and intention. A daily yoga practice may be a reset button into mindfulness and a cellular memory of no restriction and wisdom accessibility.

My practice has taught me to go deeper into my own habitual thought forms, allowing me to dissolve what is no longer working. Within this practice I have released much stored fascia memory, which when trapped, limited my access to self-truth. Therefore, yoga offers the opportunity to build greater pathways to our-self-divine and may allow one to witness oneself, having access to self-modulation, into choices favourable of ease and wellness.

In studying Sattva yoga with Rameen, a seasoned meditator since five years of age, we practice many breathing techniques—deep breath in and out, nadi shodhana (alternate nostril breathing), pranayama breathing— all of which have a connecting and settling effect on the mindbody, while expanding and unwinding coping patterns. This gives the mind something to focus on, allowing thoughts to subside. Focusing just on breathing in and out is quite enough to calm. It is an instant nervous system reset, requiring no medication, no fancy gadgets.

Yoga practice and meditation, are valuable measures and very effective in shifting oneself into a parasympathetic state, (healing rest and digest), such as the practice of Yin yoga, iRest, restorative yoga.

In Kundalini yoga there are practices, chants and movement for all emotional issues and areas in need of healing. Yet this practice can be a strong practice, and if the body is too innervated,( nervous system too exhausted), one may need to do gentle Kundalini in the beginning. The mindbody needs strength in order to support Kundalini awakening. I was blessed to attend a Kundalini ten-day retreat, on a beautiful Island in British Columbia, six months after the death of my son. *Beyond Addiction: The Yogic Path to Recovery*, was founded by Sat Dharam Kaur, ND, and integrates the work of Dr. Gabor Mate. I was humbly grateful for the gift of this practice which moved much shock and grief from the "issues in my tissues" as I witnessed in many others as well.

In *Anatomy Trains*, author Tom Meyers explains how the patterns of strain throughout the entire skeletal muscular system communicate through myofascial webbing, contributing to posture and movement compensation. His incredible work examines the interconnected web of soft tissue and the neurovascular system. Some of our largest restrictions are in the pelvic region. We hold vast amounts of emotion in the pelvic fascia; hence, a spastic digestive system. One area in our body that is constricted has an impact on the entire system including all organs and fascia which is our connective webbing. Possibly releasing these strongholds may allow us access to sovereign freedom.

A satsang, (mindful community), and practice of yoga, has been one of the greatest self-nurturing and resetting practices I have done toward wellness and joy, as it has for millions. I am grateful to the yogis everywhere, holding space, teaching tradition body-temple hygiene and conscious conductivity.

# Life-Saving Valuable Practices for Whole-Person Healing

We feel good when we participate in building a better mindbody and soul, and sharing this with the world. We feel good when we bring our energy to the present moment as children do. These are life-saving practices towards living well and staying well. When any practice is done regularly until it is our daily medicine, hearts open and mind bodies clear; we find serenity amongst the noise.

## Natural Cleansing:

Remove yourself from cellular and Wi-Fi range as much as possible, and ground and bathe in undisrupted nature.

## Massage & Bodywork:

Touch, a basic need, skin the largest receptor organ. Oh my, to feel cared for! Massage and compassionate touch have been my soul quest work and deepest passion and can be incredibly healing.

## Hydrotherapy & Hydration:

Water is sacred healing and has been used for every ailment since the beginning of time. Being well-hydrated is a matter of life and death! Float tanks are a great way to load magnesium into your systems, rebirth. Cold sunrise plunges, healing springs and rivers, bathhouses, saunas … we all have felt the healing and deep relaxation of water—from salt to sulphur we be.

*Meditation is the Divine digestion of the Cosmic Prana. The alchemy of meditation begins when the ultimate of Truth of Oneness becomes our predominate waking state awareness, and we motionlessly dance and silently sing in the sublime joy of Whole Person Enlightenment*

*~ Dr. Gabriel Cousens*

## Acupuncture:

Acupuncture works with the energy of our ever-changing body electric and organ energy meridians. Acupuncture can speed up healing tremendously. Acupuncture saved my life. Beautiful Nina, my acupuncturist took me into the womb of her home, instead of another trip to the hospital. Michael helped me move through deep grief by clearing lung and heart chi. Acupuncture is a must for anyone wanting deeper healing.

## Life Coaching:

Having a personal coach has been a complete reset in the navigation of my life. Accountability, thoughtful questioning and gentle deep listening have the potential to change the course of our journey into one of more authenticity.

## Walking:

Walking is meditative, nature is our greatest gift. To "keep my head where my feet are" as my dear friend Kelly says, is a gift we give ourselves. Walking has always been a way to release stress. The cross body movement of right arm swinging forward while left foot steps has been scientifically proven to reduce stress and connect right and left hemisphere of the brain, see (Brain Gym). When I worked in early childhood development, I used to see children who did not crawl as infants, demonstrate improved learning skills when they were given crawling and Brain Gym exercises. There is great medicine in the ancient wisdom that 30 minutes of walking per day increases healthy longevity! Walk in nature and connect.

## Chi Nei Tsang:

Otherwise known as "Unwinding the Belly," grounded into Taoism and founded by qigong doctor Mantak Chia. I have been both practitioner and student in this visceral unwinding and have found it incredibly helpful. Most of people find the belly "unknown territory."

## Reflexology:

Reflexology works on the meridians of the body through hands, feet, and ears. We are able to access the reflex points of the entire body in the sending meridian areas. Some years ago, as a student in a hands-on mastery reflexology program, I discovered something quite interesting. After an intensive weekend course, I was given homework assignments, which were due the following weekend. I spent the next week cleaning cupboards and closets and returned the following weekend not as prepared yet organized at home. My teacher laughed and delighted in saying the reflexology was working.

## Meditation:

Relaxes and resets the nervous system. Throughout this book it has been referenced how mindfulness, meditation and stress reduction lead to decreased gut-brain inflammation, and innervation due to a decrease of overstimulation and tapping into the greater whole. The importance of meditation and quieting the mind cannot be overemphasized. It is known as the core nutrient for healing. It is, in a felt sense, our way home.

## Aerobic Exercise:

One of the fastest ways to reset the nervous system, rid the body of excess cortisol, flush nitric oxide and literally "shake off" stuck energy. The Four Minute Workout by Zach Bush, is a nitric oxide releasing routine which shifts biology. Aerobic exercise decreases inflammation, turns on the brain's neurogenesis hippocampus created by brain derived neurotrophic factor (BDNF). Conscious movement and the release of stress in as little a 3–5 minutes, can oxygenize and reset the body. Disease does not like oxygen.

## Yoga / Breath-work / Laughter Yoga:

A beautiful way to reconnect, clear energy from the chakras, stimulate the meridians and become conscious of our breath, beauty, and body as one.

## Qigong / Tai Chi:

To increase good energy, release unwanted energy, increase focus and increase the ability to meditate in motion and connect cosmic orbit light with our mitochondria light.

## Hypnotherapy:

Allows us to access information that is not available to the conscious mind—aka: root/ cause issues.

## Grounding:

Otherwise known as earthing—is being barefoot in nature. It's incredibly anti-inflammatory and calming.

## Emotional Freedom Technique (EFT) & Body-talk:

This entails tapping on meridians while speaking your way through an issue, while giving yourself permission through affirmation to love yourself as you are in this moment. A powerful technique that can be use frequently with quick results.

## Silence / Nature:

Stress immediately begins to leave the energy field when we leave the business of a city and step into nature. It is essential for our well-being. Silence is the music of God.

## Cleansing / Detoxification:

Settles down mindbody inflammation quickly and quiets the "grasping" self, the nervous system and through detoxifying the bowels, we detoxify the mind.

## Story:

In interviewing a yogi regarding his understanding of the origin of when Crohn's disease came visiting, he related the practice of yoga during his time healing Crohn's disease and the breath-work and yoga practices of right mind, as being the catalyst for him rarely feeling inflamed again.

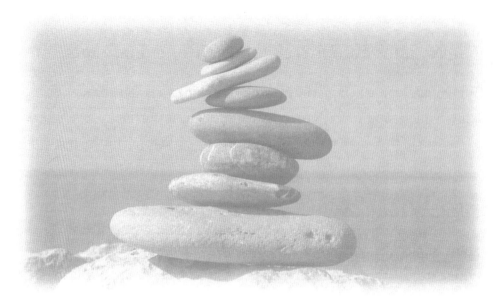

## Meditation:

Find a still quiet place within yourself.

Be open to what comes up without suppression.

Contemplate through breathing in and breathing out your life as one beautiful prayer of growth, allowing emotions to arise without judgement.

Imagine in your mind's eye all the things in your life that elevate you to a level of infinite body in mindful motion. When you soften in to yourself, allow images to come and go with breath, like ocean waves on the shore—no attachment. Allow yourself, just for a moment, to feel yourself as only energy. As you breathe in and as you breathe out.

Feel into the possibility that you are not solid matter, simply infinite energy connected to a kind and creative cosmos.

Feel yourself breathing in and out pure energy.

Tap into the oneness and the gentleness that oneness brings.

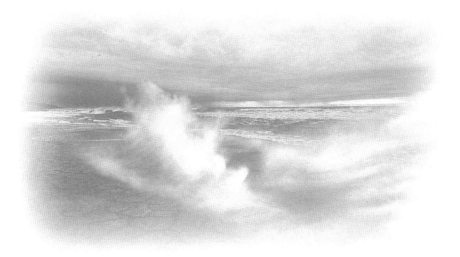

## Gratitude:

I AM infinitely grateful for my breath and the ability to take full oxygen capacity into my lungs and feed myself oxygen.
I feel the exchange and give thanks to the plant kingdom.

I AM ever so grateful that the prayers of gratitude that I send out into the universe never go unheard.
(And am reminded to be careful what I pray for!)

I AM grateful that I am able to eat and think in a way that has allowed my epigenetic blueprint to have upgraded in such a way that meditation is possible.

I AM ever so grateful for the tree-dome, plant kingdom and ocean that provides us with all the oxygen in this beautiful oxygen exchange.

I AM…

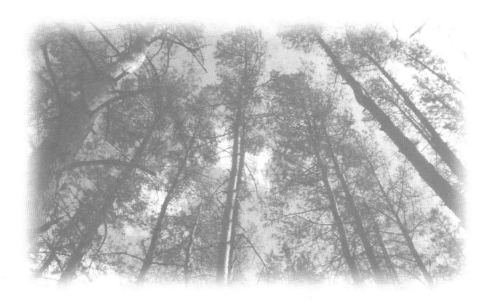

## Coming Homework:

Will you bring your awareness to deep belly-breathing throughout the day?

Meditate for even 3 minutes 3x a day.

Expand this through present moment extension of awareness —as a friend says in her simple recipe for life: "Relax…look around, relax …look around." Bringing focus to our environment, gets us out of our heads. This simple recipe relaxes the vagus nerve and stress hormones.

Will you become aware of the food and drink that brings clear and calm versus stress and adrenal overstimulation?

Gratitude and stress cannot live symbiotically—so come out of stress-fear thought and into the breathing, into an awareness of something to give thanks for, in this very moment.

# THANKSGIVING

*On Mother Earth I stand*
*Barefoot and pregnant with possibilities*
*Through my soles, I remember my soul*
*Back through ancestral twines*
*Microbial memory ALIVE*

*On Sweet Mother I kneel*
*Dandelion cleanse, a morning harvest*
*As bohemian waxwing return as ONE*
*Their unity of movement, never forgotten*
*Trees trilling of song*
*A thanksgiving sound for last year's harvest*
*A fermented fruit feast*

*On Mother Earth I lay*
*And see a time …*
*Not so far away*
*When the power of love*
*is greater than the love of power …*
*And we give thanks …*

# Chapter 3:

# What is Disease-free Health and Eating to Live?

## We are in it Together

Love is a verb. Love is inclusive and compassionate. Every generation is given the medicine to heal. I have come to know intimately, through well-researched science and witnessing others and myself heal, that our medicine is plant-food medicine that is high in water and minerals.

In Genesis 1:29 we are told of the herbs, fruit, and seeds of life to eat to remain well. We, as vertical conduits, are at the tipping point. We were raised with eating animals and their byproducts as food and convinced we need them for us to be well and strong. We are changing with Earth's biome. She is now calling us to explore the truth in the dangers in continuing what we are doing.

*The greatness of a nation and its moral progress can be judged by the way their animals are treated.*

*~ Gandhi*

Truth has always had three stages: ridicule, violent opposition and acceptance. I believe holistic plant-based nutrition' is the middle of all three, simultaneously. I feel the resistance many have in imagining themselves letting go of animals as a source of food, clothing, and entertainment.

Yet we as inhabitants of the earth are beginning to understand the suffering of one is the suffering of all, whether or not we subscribe to that. The proof is blinding.

Animals actually have greater developed senses than us humans have and the pain we have inflicted is coming back to nip us in the butt—literally and figuratively. We are back here again full circle, mutating the genes of our food so they can withstand chemical annihilation, which eats us up from the inside out. May we become hungrier for change than habits that create inflammation.

*Who are we? What is our proper role on this earth? I submit we can only begin to discover these answers if we live compassionately towards other creatures. Then peace with each other will at least be possible, as well as a deeper understanding of the mysteries of healing, freedom, and love.*

*~ **Will Tuttle***

## *Plant-Based vs Meat-Based Diet Protocols*

Studies show us that environmental factors including diet, bowel rest, and bacterial composition are worth investigation. Consideration in the implementation of whole food, plant-based diets for repair and maintenance of mindbody is worth its weight in "gold light."

*The holy four foods: fruits, vegetables, herbs and spices and wild food are more sacred and powerful because they grow from the earth and sky, enduring out in the elements day after day as they form, they are intimately connected to the forces of nature.*

***Anthony Williams** in* ***The Medical Medium***

**Lindsey Aldenberg, in Food and the Gut Microbiota in IBD, explains:** "Westernized diets rich in animal fat and protein, while low in fibre, may alter the gut microbiome in a way that may increase the risk for the development of IBD… of course, since the intestine is continually exposed to numerous antigens, a westernized diet could contain food antigens that could perpetuate the development of IBD. The authors of this systematic review concluded that high vegetable intake, high fibre and fruit intake, probiotics, was associated with decreased CD and UC risk."[10] (Aldenberg, 2012, Food and the gut microbiota in inflammatory bowel diseases: a critical connection)

A high-fat animal protein diet has been known to numb the satiate response on both a brain and gut level. What research also reveals is that it's also causing low-grade inflammation in the brain and gut, reducing sensitivity of the vagus nerve. Therefore, high animal fat diets appear to increase blood inflammatory molecules, increasing cytokines and lipopolysaccharides. With these higher amounts of animal fats, we see an increased amount of fat-inducing microbe firmicutes, which are inflammatory and often associated with higher Standard American Diets (SAD) and increased inflammation. Up to 90% of poultry and eggs are estimated to harbour pathogen bacteria such as *E.coli*.[11]

The beginning phases of the raw food diets in which I have studied at various health centres is primarily fresh organic vegetables and vegetable juicing, with rapid reduction in inflammation, intestinal bleeding and discomfort. The results of this diet was energy and normal elimination within a week, the study of one.

I continued to omit all grains, dairy, and disaccharide sugars, (fruit is an easy-to-digest monosaccharide), due to damaged villi and mucus-forming qualities.

This is what value I deemed in myself—as thousands of others achieved—on an organic whole-food, plant-based diet and bowel rest:

- Rapid drops in inflammation
- Reduction and elimination of pain
- Elevation in mood and hope
- Lengthening of telomere—yes the length of your DNA strands have shown to increase, as in the thesis work of Angela Hamlin, RN at the Tree Of Life—meaning a longer healthier life with plant medicine.

*I have come to discover that, beyond doubt,*
*what we do not eat and what we discover is eating us—*
*(stress factors, broken hearts, toxic food), are major components*
*to the health and healing of the gut.*

## Fibre & Feeding the Microbiome

Plant-based diets are highest in fibre, the prebiotic of life. This must be approached with ease and consideration with an individual who has had bowel surgery and can be resolved with juice and smoothies.

"Fibre is also important for a healthy microbiome. Some of the microbes in your gut specialize in fermenting soluble fibre, such as what's found in legumes, fruit and vegetables. Some of these fermentation byproducts also help calibrate your immune system, thereby preventing inflammatory disorders such as asthma and Crohn's disease… Other research has shown that microbes starved of fibre can begin feeding on the mucous lining of your gut, thereby triggering inflammation, which may promote or exasperate any number of diseases including ulcerative colitis."[12] (Mercola, 2016, How your gut microbiome influences your mental and physical health)

American Gut Project has collected data from over 5,000 patients who have submitted samples and dietary questionnaires. They calculated the fibre intake for various dietary groups to be: [13] (Mercola, 2016, American Gut Project)

* Paleo-like: 19 g/day
* Omnivore: 19 g/day
* Paleo: 25.1 g/day
* Omnivore, but no red meat: 27.8 g/day
* Vegetarian: 32.8 g/day
* Vegan: 43 g/day

Generally, fecal levels of protein fermentation, such as sulphide, are positively associated with protein consumption in humans. Yet evidence has shown that high dietary protein intake, including red meat, is associated with DNA damage in the colonic mucosa.[13] (Mercola, 2016, American gut project)

## The Jubilee

*There is a time*
*Not too far away*
*When we no longer fight wars*
*That don't belong to us*
*When love will feel more familiar then pain*
*And our hearts will be healed enough*
*To no longer project our wounds unto another*

*There is a time...*
*Not too far away*
*When we see blessings everywhere*
*In the water, our food, in a 'stranger's' eyes*
*When I know our children will hear more*
*kind words than any other*
*And we all know we have the power to heal*

*And we honour the POWER OF LOVE*
*Instead of the love of power*
*There is a time...*

# Eating for Peace:

## Conventional Farming, Nature Farming & "One Earth" Consciousness …

When we listen with devotion to the mindbody's higher intelligence, we become the love that we seek! Conscious-eating and conscious-gardening for peace are interwoven deeply into our cellular matrix—whispering nature's farming from sea, microbes, forests and prairies beyond. We are rapidly moving beyond genetic engineering, heavy irrigation, pesticides, deforestation and toxic fertilizers. These have become "the killing fields" of much suffering. I believe war will someday be no more.

The killing of the microbial rich "living soil" is reflected and interconnected with the destruction of our gut's microbiome—the three pounds of immunity-rich microbes that live within the crypts of our intestines—allowing us to break down, absorb, and assimilate the nutrients in our food. The introduction of genetically modified organisms (GMO) and their heavy chemical counterparts has not only destroyed our topsoil, but have also destroyed our intestines. IBD increased 40% after the introduction of GMO foods, which creates wide gaps in the villi of the intestines (leaky gut) and allows toxins to enter our entire system.

*The rich soft soil has all run away leaving the land nothing but skin and bone.*

*~ Plato*

# What Does GMO/GE Food Have to Do With It?

GMO may actually stand for "God Move Over." Both genetically engineered organisms (GEOs) and GMOs have recombinant DNA technology to alter the biochemical characteristics of an organism. In GE and GMO foods, there are three characteristics: the DNA of the plant is altered so it releases Bt toxin continuously, which paralyzes the digestive system of insects that eat it; the crop can be Roundup Ready (RR), meaning it can withstand the toxins in Roundup herbicide; and the plant can be modified to alter the genes so it is hardly recognizable by nature and God—or your body's digestive system.

GMOs are heavily toxic, create allergies, and are killing many species that connect with the GE food – bees, butterflies, insects and us! Many parents watched allergies disappear when they converted to organic food. Zen Honeycutt from *Moms Across America*, is a crusading mother bear who reversed allergies/issues in her children by committing to whole organic food. She is worthy of our attention and support. Zen reminds us moms that we buy most of the food in our households, and we must save our families from a life of illness and sick-care by making wise choices in what the family eats.

When food is modified, it allows extreme toxic spraying of Roundup that would normally kill a crop. It works on an enzymatic pathway called the shikimate pathway, which Monsanto claims is not disruptive to our health because it only affects plants and bacteria. Yet since we are mostly non-human bacteria that needs enzymatic power for everything, we are harmed through this shikimate pathway. The disruption caused by excessive use of thousands of herbicides, including Roundup, and the GMO alteration of the plant results in excessive growth of orange moulds. These release mycotoxins contaminate feeds that have been documented to cause spontaneous abortions and other reproductive harm in livestock. These additional toxins are implicated in cancers and other problems in humans as well as livestock.

**As Dr. Zach Bush explains:**

"We're washing all that glyphosate or Roundup right into our gutters and into our municipal water systems. The huge problem with Roundup or glyphosate is that it's extremely water-soluble, which means it's going to stay in the water systems throughout the ecosystem. You fast-forward to today where we're using one and a half billion pounds of that antibiotic worldwide. And it's interesting because it's never been patented as a weed killer. That's what they tell us it is but, in fact, it's an antibiotic. It was patented as an antibiotic, anti-fungal, anti-parasitic. It blocks an important enzyme pathway called the shikimate pathway. This enzyme pathway produces the ring or aromatic amino acids. There are only twenty-six amino acids. Three that Round up blocks is phenylalanine, tyrosine and tryptophan—all three of those are critical for brain function and are probably the most critical for brain health."[6] (The Rich Roll Podcast, March 18, 2018)

Yet plants are becoming Roundup resistant and through conscious reconnection to our land, chemical farming may be on its way out. May we begin biodynamic and effective microorganism practices, as the "cure" for dis-ease and the medicine to illuminate our way home.

In August 2018, Monsanto suffered a major blow with a jury ruling that the company was liable for a terminally ill man's cancer, awarding him $289M in damages and opened the door for many lawsuits to follow.

Dwayne Johnson, a 46-year-old former grounds-keeper, won a huge victory in the landmark case with the jury determining that Monsanto's Roundup weed-killer caused his cancer and that the corporation failed to warn him of the health hazards from exposure. The jury further found that Monsanto "acted with malice or oppression." [14]

The documentary Genetic Roulette—*The Gamble of Our Lives and the book Seeds of Deception*, both by consumer activist Jeffrey Smith, reveal some of the damage created from GMO Roundup Ready food in the following summary: gut permeability, neurological damage (GMO animals display autism), and illness across the board. Mr. Smith has documented that "inflammatory Bowel Disease (IBD) increased 40% immediately after the introduction of GMO, and gut/brain issues rose at alarming rates; autopsied livestock that consumed GMO feed have shown completely destroyed intestines; very high rate of newborn animal mortality; and spinal, genital and gut deformities." Many documentaries, peer reviews and investigative books have followed this one.[73]

Michael Fox, a respected humane veterinarian, has discovered all skin and gut problems in pets, including itching, aggression and tumours relating to digestive issues, usually clear up when they are given organic, non-GMO food.

Autopsies on GMO-fed animals showed complete disintegration of intestinal lining as well as ulcerated livers after two years. The Bt-toxin glyphosate and other crazy synergistic chemicals in Roundup break open the insides of insects. It does the same in people. An allergen is something the immune system sees as foreign: GMOs are foreign invaders. It's not surprising that autoimmune and inflammatory diseases skyrocketed after Roundup Ready crops were introduced. There is much evidence indicating that glyphosate interferes with critical chemicals, amino acids and nutrient availability, creating deficiencies in plant food and, ultimately, in humans. This is a really big deal! Just look around at how poorly we are feeling and sleeping, with hormone disruptors and nutrient-empty food.

Glyphosate research that is not funded by agri-chemical companies tells us the herbicide increases the ability for pathogens to develop antibiotic resistance by disrupting the gut bacteria along with manganese and other valuable nutrients essential for our wellness and immunity.

Glyphosate was originally patented in China as an antibiotic, but deemed harmful and unusable because of its numerous negative side effects. An antibiotic with negative side-effects on our food …yikes! Immunity becomes very weak without the beneficial bacteria and rich diversity of minerals needed in our foods, and organisms, like us, who eat these plants become prone to pathogenic fungi, viruses and bacteria, just the same as the weak mineral deficient plant develops into. This is the EarthGut connection.

**Glyphosate may be on its way out due to public advocacy, so let us be wise to not let them slip in another chemical as dangerous, in its' place!**

Look at how many humans are turning to probiotics because the bacteria essential to our health have been annihilated from our soil, our food, and our medicine. According to the World Health Organization, 99% of us are deficient in minerals since we wiped out our amazing nutrient-dense topsoil, beginning over 100 years ago and escalating over the past few decades.

Much of the food we eat is no longer medicine. Chemical farming is starving, not feeding the world due to its ridiculously weak nutrient value and its ability to wipe out good microbes, allowing pathogens to get a stranglehold on our digestion. Our guts rely heavily on bacteria synthesis, nutrient and enzymatic action, that our beautiful human biology once knew how to make so naturally when we ate from living soil.

The reduction of living soil is on a scale never seen before by humankind. When the soil is gone, so are we. Insensitive chemical farming has contributed to the soil ecosystems' loss of diversity and microbial presence at an alarming rate. This type of farming does not respect or acknowledge the symbiosis of nature or the patterns of Mother Earth and her revitalizing resting periods. For proof, just look around at the epidemics of health issues that have arisen since the introduction of GMO crops and the rise in gut issues at the core of all these!

The wind will carry GMO pollen for thousands of miles. In both the United States and Canada, 98% of GMO food is not labelled and many foods are irradiated to kill living bacteria without our knowledge. This is changing! People, when informed, naturally gravitate toward non-GMO food. Much food is irradiated, destroying enzymes and vitamins such as, B, C, E, and K vitamins and all medicinal properties of food, herbs and spices. In Canada I have some precious food co-ops which supply bulk non-irradiated herbs for my food medicine. These are the reason we are given for irradiating food by *Canadian Food and Safety Inspection*:

- **To reduce microbial load on spices and dehydrated seasoning preparations, meaning it destroys bacteria, moulds and yeast which cause food to spoil.**
- **To control insects in wheat, flour and whole wheat flour.**
- **To increase shelf life by preventing sprouting or germination in potatoes and onions.**
- **Again this is, the war on living food and food as medicine omits the truth; sprouting food and using bacteria for assisting us in absorbing nutrients is key.**

**This following, from biologist Sheryl McCumsey, trailblazer for Pesticide-Free Alberta, is an invitation to find mindful EarthGut practices:**

"Chances are, if you are reading this book, you have already opened a door to the reality that what goes into your body will impact several functions of your body. It is not such a hard concept to grasp, but one in which many people seem to have seriously disconnected from. We know that clean air versus polluted air has a profound impact on our health. How about our food? We take medicine to address disease. We rarely consider the cause of disease.

Science is the work of observation. However, we all have confirmation bias, meaning "a bias that confirms one's pre-existing beliefs or hypotheses." (re:wiki). How do we break though bias that may be influenced by things we do not admit to ourselves? Are we doing ourselves a disservice?

Pesticides are used to kill things, and they are effective until they become resistant. They are poisons, not inert substances. This is why we do have warnings on labels for these products. What is interesting is that weeds and insects develop resistance to pesticides and we continue to focus on finding yet another poison in order to destroy them. Like disease, we do not consider why they are there—or if our approach to this is simply based in the wrong direction? Prevention of disease is all about creating good health. Are we doing this with agriculture?

Where people tend to disagree is how powerful and harmful a pesticide is. Folks argue that Health Canada registers it so it must be "safe." A good doctor is also concerned with drug interactions, same with pharmacists. They are aware that side effects can and do outweigh benefits.

The attitude is very different with pesticides. We mix them up and do not test the synergistic impacts. We also do not even test "products." Any chemist understands that reactions of different chemicals matter. The real world is not a laboratory and it is very difficult to study how a pesticide impacts the environment, which is variable. Animal studies have limitations. Rats possess enzymes to process poisons that we do not have. This is where epidemiology becomes important to study and control health-related diseases and problems.

Health Canada does not have any laboratories of its own and it is only very recently that a couple of epidemiologists have been added to staff there. Without looking at the impacts being found in medical studies such as these, our regulatory agency is missing very important data. Currently there are 7,000 pesticide products on the market.

Canadians are suffering the consequences. We have some of the highest levels of gut diseases in the world found in the very young. People who immigrate to Canada become sick. All of this is also illustrated in studies and often we hear about antibiotic exposure or environmental impacts as a possible cause. People who get sick may go on drugs and find they are not that effective.

The federal audit of the Pest Management Regulatory Agency came out in the fall of 2015. In this audit, they discussed how eighty pesticides have "conditional registrations." What this means is that we have pesticides on the market, in our food system, on our land, found in the water and being fed to our children without the required science submitted. If you are not consuming organic food, you are consuming pesticides that have not been assessed.

In addition, we do not test products like Roundup as a whole, which has a much higher toxicity than glyphosate as illustrated in studies (up to a 1,000 times).

As well, chlorpyrifos, which is mentioned in exhibit 1.4 of the audit, has not been properly re-evaluated since registration in 1969. There are 2,000 peer-reviewed studies on this very potent and persistent neurotoxic pesticide that shows there is no safe exposure and can result in long-term impairments in working memory, IQ, lower body weight, and possibly ADHD as well as autism.

As individuals, we have the power to choose what we consume, which is a very powerful thing we can do for our own health and for the health of the planet. We depend on this planet to sustain us. We can choose to ignore these concerns and connections by paying the price of poor health later on OR we can collaborate with the change makers and transform our own health at the same time."[15] (McCumsey, 2019, An essay on pesticide free Canada)

Getting connected to growing food and earthing is critical in times like these. The problem with chemicals, pesticides, fertilizers and herbicides is that they kill the microbial colonies in the soil, disrupt the natural patterns of nature, prevent nutrient uptake for plants from the soil, and poison the water table and water cycle. They are systemic and absorbed into the food supply to be consumed by us. There is a vicious cycle, once pesticides, herbicides and fertilizers are introduced, more and more chemicals are required to achieve the same results and eventually the soil becomes toxic rendering it lifeless and useless. Microbes, living soil, and the *compassion cure* are our escape routes.

Many of these chemical compounds do not break down quickly in the environment. These pesticides are toxic at every test level: they damage insect, avian and aquatic life, as predicted in Rachel Carson's *Silent Spring,* disrupting nature's pattern. An example of this is that birds are natural pest eradicator and if they eat insecticide laced bugs they or their young are adversely affected.

Precipitation (e.g., rainfall) samples have significant levels of glyphosate in them as do our waterways. There is so much Roundup in our environment that it is falling from the skies. The further disconnection from the land, the more we have been able to spray heavy chemicals and alter nature such as in GMOs.

Just because our doctors, friends, and community are not necessarily talking about this, does not mean it does not exist or will go away. Silencing truth is not the answer; speaking truth is our conscious way out.[15]

# *The Antidote to Conventional Farming:*

- Eating and growing organic/veganic/biodynamic plant-based, whole-food only—for both animals and people, usually comes with huge health benefits. This is true for myself.

- Reclaiming living topsoil is key! So why is energizing the topsoil so important for civilization? If we look into the archaeological records, many large cities that have experienced soil degradation and the collapse of local food supplies were no longer able to support urban populations, as we are—WE ARE THE EARTH! Knowing this is key to our protection of living soil and species diversity.

- Most of the microbial action and the living roots of our plants are in the first 10 inches of the substrate. Plants need substantial living soil in order to have proper uptake of nutrients. This living soil and diversity is the greatest contributor to pest control. Most social disease, beginning with gut health, and has a way of curing itself if the terrain is favourable.

- Effective Microorganisms is Kuan Yin's gift for gardening for Peace and God's antidote is to restore.

- Living an uncontaminated food and probiotic-rich life.

- Detox therapy daily—deep hydration, infra saunas, lymph brushing, Zach Bush 4 Minute Workout, rebounding, fasting, juicing, exercise, sleeping, sound therapy. Healthy soil helps us remember our divine essence.

- Ayurveda teaches that disease begins when we are imbalanced, and in disharmony with our environment, five senses, and beyond. When balance is disrupted, our body weakens. In an imbalanced environment, pathogens thrive, muscles contract, and energy flows within the body are significantly disrupted. Through Ayurveda, we balance all elements of our environment within the equilibrium of spice, herb, oil, scent, and plant medicine; along with bringing in beauty through all senses, especially through deep-sensory healing of massage and herbal nutrition.

# *Nature Farming*

Nature farming practices, respect the land and all creatures, while using natural re-mineralization thought techniques such as EM, sea minerals, rock dust, etc.

Nature farming began in 1935 with Mokichi Okada in Japan. The philosophy was to create agricultural ecosystems that harmonized and respected nature through minimal disturbance. This type of practice proved to have kept disease in check and allowed the soil to heal itself.

*The basis of Nature Farming is an appreciation for the power of "living soil," which is the key factor that makes the system sustainable and resilient.*

*~ Dr. Gabriel Cousens*

The use of natural compost and the application of EM was founded by Dr. Higa in 1969. EM was brought to the Tree of Life in 1998 by John Phillips. In his *Gardening for Peace*, he says nature farming is designed by our higher power:

"Practical tools employed include microbial inoculants such as EM, beneficial insects, organically grown seeds (Non-GMO) cover crops and green manure, weed suppressive cover crops and mechanical cultivation, flame weeding, compost and organic fertilizers, rock dust, minimal tillage, greenhouses and other advanced technologies of eco-farming… EM is a consortium of beneficial microorganisms comprised of five main groups: photosynthetic bacteria, lactic acid bacteria, beneficial yeast, beneficial fungi and actinomycetes."[16] (Phillips, 2019)

Civilization has always been only as healthy as its topsoil. Veganic gardening as developed at the Tree of Life Centre in Patagonia, Arizona, USA, uses EM to create a model of probiotic farming based on "living soil." It omits all use of animal products for fertilizer and production inputs. This allows us some protection against bacteria/viruses, such as *E. coli* and GMO toxins.

Veganic nature farming works symbiotically with nature's law—one mind, one earth, one people. It is based on the understanding that the personal is political: how we do something is how we do everything, and the karmic effect of taking care of the whole and the deep peace that accompanies this.

Working with nature, enriching soil with EM, sea minerals, and other earth practices may very well heal our guts, hearts, and brains. A diet rich in both prebiotic and probiotic living vegan food is possibly our only way home. Living soil equals living whole. What is happening in this time in history is a major food revolution. The state of your soil is a direct reflection of the state of our culture–what is happening on the macro-scale of mono crop conventional farming is reflecting throughout the entire planet with the significant loss of diversity.

As I write this book, I lightly participate within a conscious community of hemp farmers. I create the nutrition piece of green hemp powder and food, while others are harvesting the stems, hearts, buds/leaves and seed for the use in everything including CBD medicine (without THC). Hemp has few insect pests and every bit is usable. A beloved community is going to begin the creation of hempcrete tiny homes on my land in the spring. Others are pressing amazing omega hemp oils and hearts, sensations I savour in my kind kitchen. We get by with a little help from our friends on our way to happiness and eco-love.

Humic and fulvic acid are often used to heal the gut. When terrahydrite in *ION\*Bione* is established in the gut, it strengthens the gut lining against glyphosate.

*Regenerative soil practices,*
*nature farming and*
*self-love shared,*
*are our way home.*

*~Tami Hay*

# I feel the Earth move under my feet!

Grounding or earthing has been known to be one of the most anti-inflammatory and effective methods of healing. Clint Ober, author of *Earthing*, shares this knowledge with passion in his earthing movement. Appreciating this earth-awakening movement;connecting the dots, through a multitude of discussions and courses, documentaries and sharing circles, farmers and spirit keepers around the globe.

Ancients are calling us back to remember. Walk barefoot, meditate and mediate real-plant medicine as much as possible, and re-collect sweet remembrance.

*"When we eat,*
*we are biting into the*
*living planet.*
*If our eating process is not based on*
*love and compassion,*
*all of our other actions*
*are bound to suffer."*

~ ***Dr. Gabriel Cousens***

## A prayer to the Divine:

*Sweet Creator, with heartfelt divinity*
*May you quiet me?*
*Guide me*

*Shelter me and lift me*
*Releasing all swords of superiority and righteousness*

*May it be done on Earth as it is in Heaven?*
*Violence toward all sentient beings*
*forever put to rest*
*In the name of Love*

*And so it is....*

Conscious eating, our digestive health and conscious gardening go together, understanding the beauty in connecting to the food we are growing. Highly mineralized, electrolyzed sun-food equals energy. Live sun-food has the most life force and when we grow this food ourselves or support local organic/veganic family farms, the freshness contributes to the nutritional value for us.

Natural permaculture methods respect all life forms; our interdependence with swamp lands, forests, and all the naturally occurring mulch, etc. that contribute to living soil. Nature farming acknowledges natural patterns, seasons and all life force.

A fresh and holistic way of thinking and doing, that puts our ecology and cosmos at the centre, may be our only possible way out of our global crisis. By eradicating all animal food produced through fear, cruelty and suffering, we are clearing the same discord from our energy field and beyond. This is a very important truth to remember and we may be on a new frontier of self understanding and empowerment.

I was attending a Native sweat lodge ceremony some 16 years ago, long before "vegan" entered my energy field. A woman beside me declined the wild meat stew. She explained to me eating meat overstimulated her and she could feel the adrenaline and fear running through her veins that the animal felt while it was being hunted and dying. I thought, *A little woo woo she is!*

Years later, after refraining from eating meat for some time and then having some, I experienced the same thing—unsettled and agitated. I later learned in the astounding book *Spiritual Nutrition* eating anxiety-laden animals and has a stimulating effect on the body. Dr. Zach Bush now speaks to his patients of such matters—the connection between anxiety and eating animals that have endured great suffering.

Waking up to truth is "coming to," if you will. When we eat in a way that clears our 72,000 Nadis—we GET IT!! The awakening is like the peeling of an onion—the cleaner we eat and think, the deeper our awareness and sensitivity becomes towards toxins, disharmony, and disorder. We may lose our appetite for distraction and gain a taste for peace. The addiction of denial may loosen its grip and begin to fall away.

*We may begin to see that the Holistic Food revolution is no longer a matter of choice, it is a matter of survival. I believe the restlessness of the world chaos is our unconscious demanding LIGHT. Right knowledge into action is power.*

The compassion and truth we now extend matters. Holistic is not about abstaining from stuff we enjoy. I have inspired so very many in my kitchen with amazing easy-to-prepare and really tasty cuisine! My heart sings as we creatively begin to love food that loves us back. It becomes about compassionate action, loosening the restraints of cultural forgetting, and living and nourishing the world in a way that includes peace, love and healthy microbes for all.

Throughout the last decade of research towards understanding wellness following an IBD diagnosis, story-after-story emerged of people who have completely healed all symptoms of IBD through an organic and veganic plant-based diet.

One of the earliest, most effective diets for me in the beginning stages of CD was a natural hygiene diet based on predigested fruit and juice smoothies, green juice, fasting, elemental diets, and rest. One of my favourites was celery juice blended with bananas for electrolyte replenishing. I studied the works of doctors of natural hygiene and was able to correlate the single most causative effect on IBD: eating the diet our Western society heavily promotes. The body, at this stage, has difficulty digesting fat as the liver enzymes are often depleted. (See more on diet and bowel rest in the Appendix of this book).

Most people with IBD also have *Mycobacteria,* such as overgrowth of *Candida.* This must be considered in the healing food protocol.

Animal products are acid and mucus forming, high in unhealthy fat, void of fibre and water content and incredibly high in pathogenic bacteria. People with IBD want to avoid animal products because they tax our digestive system and putrefy an already sluggish bowel, which produces pathogenic bacteria as a toxic by-product.

When we cook fats and starches at a high temperature, they produce free radicals, known as acrylamides, that are indigestible and extremely toxic to the body. Many of us people with IBD are told to cook our food and to avoid fiber. In the early stages, with the colon ulcerative and raw, an elemental diet of liquid and predigested foods allows the body and bowels to rest.

When a person suffering with IBD or IBS has inflammation of the mucosa lining, the villa (finger-like projections covering the digestive tract that helps break down complex carbohydrates) are usually flattened and damaged. Gottschall's diet, which she discovered through research in her "mother bear" attempt to heal her dying child of colitis, also included meat and fermented dairy products. The problem being is 75% of people are allergic to dairy. It is not just the lactose (milk sugar) that is eaten during the fermenting process; it is also the massive protein molecule in milk that is designed to make a baby calf grow to 600 pounds within two years. The pathogens in milk have often been the culprit of salmonella poisoning and most dairy cows are not treated humanely.

It was when I went organic plant-based that I was able to experience the profound and significant healing in my recovery as is true for many who have taken this path to healing. The beginning phases were fresh organic vegetables with a small amount of fruit juicing for often a month at a time. I had smoothies, often made from celery and banana, and sometimes soft monosaccharide food such as mashed squash for the more emotionally satisfying meal later in the day.

We are ALL weakened by the heavy chemicals and pesticides sprayed on food and tilled into our soil, grasses, wetlands and leaking into the water table and air. How could we not be? I have seen many people heal environmental allergen and gut problems when their internal environment was cleaned up and strengthened. I have seen many heal by just turning to local and organic food. Even the slightest ingestion of a sensitivity-food can keep our chronic feedback loop of internal inflammation alive. The fact that we have no choice but to breath in glyphosate is a world gone mad! It puts much more emphasis on us to be extra kind and "knowledge rich" with our health.

Most toxins are fat-soluble, but not glyphosate. Its water-soluble poison can move freely through the once-tight junctions of our colon's single-cell protection and easily cross the blood-brain barrier. This is scary stuff. In order to heal, we must change everything we are doing back into the grassroots of honouring food medicine and reconnecting through the lens of ancient microbes.

How do we return to nature? Maybe, just maybe, our mitochondria are looking for our missing microbes, our natural way of nourishment, and the diverse bacteria that are rejuvenated through re-inoculation, light and natural hygiene.

Some say that when we try to break Mother Nature, she will break us. Is it because we have separated ourselves from her laws that we are in a global health crisis? Is gut inflammation the STOP sign—red, agitated and right in front of our mouths?

*I have come to discover that, beyond doubt, what we do not eat and what we discover is eating us, are the major components to our health.*

## GMO Free Are We

*Glyphosate, DDT, Dioxin*
*You are gone*
*Leaving, leaving*

*Wake up, shake it up people!*
*Eat, Pray, Live!*
*We are One!*
*We're talking about a revolution*
*Ancients and*
*Earth Peace keepers …*
*Gathering. . .*

*One day we said to our land*
*'I want to be your friend'*
*And everything changed. . .*
*Chains fell, thunder roared, the earth moved*
*She had to shake us up, wake us up*

*An awakening is upon us*

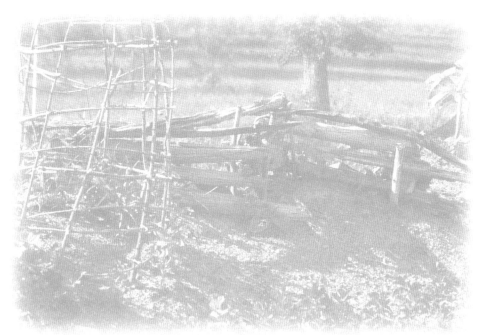

## Meditation:

Lie on Earth, resting your tired adrenals as she supports you. Begin awareness of breath, feeling yourself sinking into her microbial-rich land. Stay with her pulse …allowing it to become yours.

Find a quiet place within, bringing awareness from feet to head, while releasing tension in each area.

Now feel the joy and the microbial upgrade that having a dog, or spending time in nature, brings to our microbiome.

Imagine for a moment you can let go of the false "truth" that you cannot thrive on plants alone.

Imagine filling your life with the joy of growing and sharing live plant food in all its many forms.

Sit in your peace garden as long as you wish, listening to the birds and the sounds of this living orchestra. Let it become you.

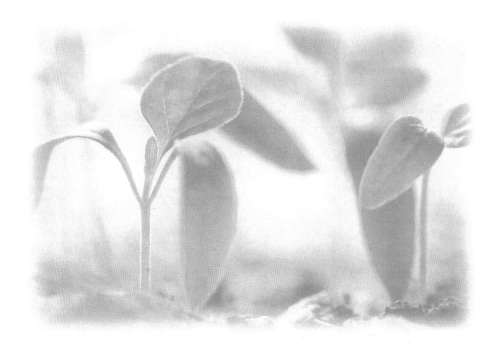

## Gratitude:

I AM grateful we are ONE; and the knowing of this as I cultivate it in my outer and inner garden.

I AM grateful for all the dedicated people, doctors and mentors who have helped us understand that a plant-powered life is both a compassionate act towards us and a gift to all sentient beings and ONE planet

I AM …

## Coming Homework:

Will you begin a new relationship with food, finding local farmers, markets, shops, community gardens?

Will you join Farmer Footprints?

Read: GutBliss, The World Peace Diet, The Medical Medium, and Conscious Eating.

Journal about the root of compassion and what sentient beings this should include.

Watch the documentaries Earthlings and Cowspiracy

Join a community and Moms Across America

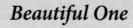

## Beautiful One

It's time to fast,
A new season is upon you,
A new Moon, a new view,
In your busy-ness
You are leaving your "Holy Rhythm,"
And everything is getting too fast, you're eating,
talking and walking

It is time to fast, Sacred One
For it is time to rest, reset, and remember. . .

And I shall poureth unto you
in the sweet, sweet emptiness.

# Chapter 4:

## *Fasting & Bowel Rest:*
## *Hydration &*
## *Commitment Healing*

Bowel cleansing and rest is the first protocol to reducing inflammation, bowel toxicity and pain fast! Intestinal toxemias contribute to mental disorders and diseases.

- What does fasting for health and spiritual benefits mean exactly?
- Why and when do you fast and how do you do this safely?

I wish to begin this chapter honouring the fact that many people struggle with eating disorders. Fasting is a great way to reset, yet for many, it may trigger compulsive thoughts from past eating disorders. If one has had past issues such as this, please consult your doctor, consider stabilizing eating patterns and seek counsel and support instead of considering a fast.

Fasting is the absolute "fast-track" for releasing bowel toxicity quickly, turning on anti-inflammatory pathways and, when juicing, an amazing way to begin re-hydrating with structured water from pure raw veg / fruit. Indican tests, which are marker tests that examine bowel toxicity, indicate that on a seven-day green juice cleanse, all bowel toxicity is gone, and genes and epigenetic health markers are significantly upgraded.

# Emotional Readiness

Fasting from ANYTHING that has a negative impact on oneself and, therefore, the health of "ALL," is of benefit. We can fast from all-solid food, surrendering of habitual eating with an intention that includes making space from the world, reconnecting and ending the fast feeling closer to divine energy, inspiration, self control and our true nature.

Fasting truly is the "fast-track" to healing. But when you have used food to comfort as I have, it is important to seek support!

As far as mental health goes, it is essential to go into a fast understanding the psychosocial connection with food habits, our tribe, and our communities. This is why it may be helpful to remove oneself from all distraction (cell phone addiction, mass media, negative depleting practices, places and things) in order to heal the mental-emotional-physical body. We may then begin to build mental microbiome health on clear waters, in a biogenetic biosphere of love.

Fasting can allow us to transcend and dissolve the shackles of past emotional, physical and spiritual pain of known and unknown origin. Simply put, fasting, if done correctly, has the potential to heal unhealthy patterns.

For myself, when I was unable to eat and was wasting away in a dark spiral called IBD, juicing and receiving maximum nutrition through a deep hydration protocol, without the fibre, was of incredible benefit and helped me regain my health.

Fasting has the ability to help heal the root cause of addictive patterning right from the beginning of the "utero addictive brain." Stimulating food and drink—salt, sugar and fat at high amounts

—is like brain cocaine, and we have difficulty putting them down. They zing us out of our emotional body when the feeling seems too overwhelming. Juicing and fasting allows us to rest into what emerges.

What is in the way is "us." This works with the vulnerable us that uses substances to cope. Many of us are born and bathed in utero, with juices of stressed parents who had to cope with unimaginable circumstances. Blood and biochemical alterations occur due to food, caffeine, alcohol, and nicotine (remember the commercials with a doctor blowing smoke into a baby's face to prove smoking was safe) and now we are beginning to see the results our diet's impact has on disease and our digestion.

Knowledge can give rise to both power and compassion. Grace is divine and intention is sweet. Beginning a fast with the intention to be still and support a quiet mind has the potential to create spaciousness for the coming and going of attachments and cravings of substances. Through mindfulness, we may allow grasping to fall away. This is the calling to "be in the world, not of it."

One thing does lead to another. I have realized only one over-stimulating choice can lead to a cascade of others as one serving of sugar can begin sugar cravings. We cannot feed our addictive brain and listen deeply to our bodies at the same time. There does come a time when the old skin must be shed. There is a saying "how we do something is how we do everything." This transition to better health of mindbody may take years and we are invited to be gentle with ourselves. Peace is the point and end goal. From a loving, kind heart and deeper self-love, we will be able to give light, not heat. Fasting is an ancient proven practice. In various interviews I have had with fasters, many of them expressed how they were divinely guided during the fast to live out their dharma, (life-purpose or calling) in ways they were not previously aware of.

**Story:**

Rachel Solomon, founder of *Optimum Health Institute,* was one who found her spiritual guidance. I was told her epiphany to open up *Optimum Health Institute* based on Ann Wigmore's *Hippocrates Health Institute* came to her during her first fast.

Getting to the root of inflammation is essential. Resetting our mindbody with fasting is essential.

## Fasting Is Most Likely As Old As Eating. Why Should One Fast?

- ❦ To reset EVERYTHING from addictions. To our pace and outward focus: reset epigenetic, genetic, and nutrigenomic imprints; bring peace to situations.

- ❦ Self-control building; to begin today because tomorrow never comes; to remember why we are here.

- ❦ To heal the root cause of diseases—dehydration, toxemia, over-acidification and inflammation, which leaves us enervated and exhausted. Our digestive power is weak during inflammation; fasting allows it to heal.

- ❦ Fasting empowers, renews and strengthens self-trust and divine dharma.We literally build a new beginning. Fasting is the quickest way to turn on the glutathione, anti-aging genes if done while using a re-hydration protocol.

  In summary, Dr. Gabriel Cousens tells us: "Fasting increases our spiritual connection from the frenzy of life and is a tremendous reset;

creates a quieter mind; opens doors to the Divine; reconnects us with our life purpose; resets our Holy Rhythm; and is used to heal all disease in the four aspects of detox–physical, emotional, spiritual and mental. Therefore it is safer to fast outside the city in a supported environment while upgrading our epigenetic program of dopamine and endorphin-opioid-like substances and resetting disease states. Fasting refines the mind, refines the emotions, elevates the spirit, upgrades you back to a normal physiology." Robert Young in the book *Sick and Tired* says we are 'alkaline by design' and the pH effect of cleansing the blood by juicing has miraculous results. He says juicing is always his foundation because juicing unblocks elimination organs; and since all functions of the body produce waste, we must continue cleaning, clearing and building new cells in order to maintain health in an unhealthy world.

## *When Does Fasting Begin?*

The beginning phases of fasting allow a much-needed physiological rest to the digestive system, resetting outward focus and addictive tendencies. This is the difference between a spiritual fast and not eating: when you remove yourself from habituation and go inward and upward while remaining deeply grounded to Earth. At day three, a purification process known as "autolysis" or "auto digestion" begins. In day two and three, fasting moves from glucose to fat metabolism, signalling the fast has begun and we are increasing our ability to rid the body of dying cells.

*"The body draws energy by decomposing and burning unused substances and metabolic waste with the help of bacteria and enzymes. This is the important part of fasting: breaking down superfluous tissue mobilizing the toxins from stored areas." Mirabel Arizpe*

Dr. Gabriel Cousens' indicant test for bowel toxicity, done after a fast, reveals the toxins are usually 100% gone on day six or seven on a green juice cleanse. He says fasting allows us to see how it builds prana faster when the body is cleared from the constant spasm of inflammation. Therefore, fasting and the building of prana allows our hearts to be more open to life—clearing habits and emotional residue that keep us chronically inflamed. These circulating toxins may cause headaches, nausea, halitosis and emotional arising, and then be gone! "Autolysis is the process of the body digesting its own cells. In the body's wisdom, it selectively decomposes those cells and tissues which are in excess, diseased, damaged, aged or dead."[11]

Fasting is not starving. It is a discipline on the way to the Beyond. Starvation occurs only when the body has used up all its reserves. If one is already depleted from IBD, at this time soft fruit such as organic non-GMO papaya and bananas may be a lifesaver. The body's wisdom will always eat up the 'rubbish' first. Often the sign of returned hunger or the sign of the body eating muscle is a good indication a fast should stop—GENTLY.

Many people with IBD are already wasting away. This may be where an elemental diet can be included. I am not referring to Ensure, a high-fructose, corn syrup-filled, empty nutrition replacement. I suggest a banana smoothie blended with organic celery juice.

A safe bet is always a seven-to-ten-day juice fast, watered down if one has diarrhea, and/or elemental smoothies. In this way, the body's minerals will not be further depleted. Fasting gives the body a chance to catch up to its job of excreting as it removes toxins from tissue and causes the body to use up excess fat. I have known people to heal colitis by living on juiced vegetables, hydrating water, and fruit smoothies until complete healing occurred.

*Bring to the fire*
*All that no longer shines*
*Bring to the fire*
*Your worries, burdens, baggage*
*And we together "will burn the rubbish"*
*From your bowels, blood, bones*

*What is happening—you ask, while Autolysis breaks down to rebuild*
*As waste debris*
*Sets you free?*

*We move from prebirth to rebirth*
*For us, our children and the Next Seven Generations unseen.*

# How Do We Fast With Ease?

This is challenging for many. Many people have used food for everything other than hunger for so very long, and the thought of letting go of this security blanket sends them into panic. After body wasting and literally starving with IBD, I have come to greatly appreciate the support of community, time away to be still, and rejuvenation centres. I recommend this to everyone, for its support and resonant energy of trust.

## There are many ways to also support ourselves:

- We drink pure water and electron green drinks
- Sleep sleep and sleep more to restore
- Move the body
- Rest and breathe
- Yoga
- Journal
- Feel emotions
- Sit in a tree
- Walk, pray, meditation
- Enzymes
- Zeolite, fasting elixirs, iodine, fulvic and humic acid, ION*Bione
- Enemas
- Massage, please have healthy touch to soothing your soul
- NATURE walking barefoot
- Connect with others on the same journey
- Laugh
- Educate ourselves
- SELF-LOVE!

*Start at the root of your misaligned emotions, Sweet One,*
*THE INTESTINES.*
*In the seventh day*
*You will no longer have to try so hard to be 'positive'*

*Come back ever so gently*
*With purified LOVE*
*As if feeding your Beloved baby*
*For you have reset your telomeres and your fears*

*Let the back bends, Mother Earth walk and water,*
*your smile*
*give you energy*

*Follow the light, the Ancients*
*Lay down the tattered swords of worn-out habits*
*You are protected*

*Go deep, deeper still*
*Into the roots*

*Be your own Watch-master observing the beyond*
*The ebb and flow and the come and go*
*Of desires, craving, emptiness*
*Back into the nothingness*

*For everything passes my child*

*Go into the beyond,*
*Far beyond Hungry Ghosts*

*Come all Beings tattered and tempted*
*Come into triumph and fast for freedom*

*The days when play, sunshine, butterflies and wide-open*
*skies were your daily feasts*

*And remember …*

*When you really let go of the refrigerator door or the next meal*
*You will floweth over with unexpected delight*
*Into the sweetness of the stomach's emptiness.*

When researching and working with many people with dis-ease, it was clear emotional hunger was often a common emptiness felt. Therefore, it is best to not try to fit into any fasting mould. Instead, begin with a hydration protocol and a hydrating pure organic diet, nice and low on the food chain.

Yes, it is respect, right action and Divine timing in everything, Szekely in the book, *Essene Science of Fasting*, says it is often best for people to begin with a one- or two-day fast and continue right living building up from there. And so we breathe, deeper and more aware, exhaling fear back into the nothing. We breathe in gratitude for this oxygen and water gifts, as they aid the oxidation of harmful waste from all organs and tissue.

Nature has an incredible way of integrating spiritual fasting. This morning I jumped out of bed, as I watched the morning sun illuminate the snowcapped mountain peaks. The heaviness of my mind the night before vanished into this vast sweet wilderness!

*May fasting bring all sentient beings to happiness and freedom*
*May fasting free the shackles of addiction and mind-trappings*
*May fasting bring all Beings health, peace and non-causal joy and love*

(See much more on fasting how-to's and many recipes in the Appendix)

## Meditation:

Sit quietly and breathe deeply into the belly's emptiness.

Connect with the infinite space that is the truth of YOU.

Breathe deeply and welcome all that arises from this infinite space of pure emptiness brimming with infinite potential.

Breathe deeply and welcome all that arises from the infinite spaces within every empty space of you.

As you connect with this infinite emptiness invite the paradox of brimming fullness of your source, your soul, and your life force to play into this space.

Continue to breathe and source your own soul, your own wisdom and your true nature inside, as this emptiness reconvenes with the unknown you.

Invite this brimming emptiness into and through each cell of your being and your microbiome.

Be curious what is here to emerge.

Be curious what gifts are awaiting you in the emptiness.

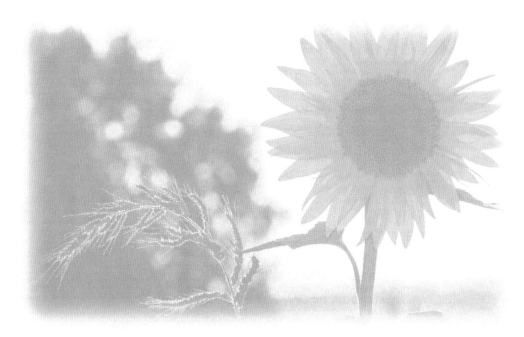

## Gratitude:

I AM grateful for the energy, clarity and re-activation of my soul's purpose through fasting.

I AM grateful for understanding during a fast that I have more energy and that energy comes from so many forms other than food—breath, water, nature, yoga, prayer, meditation.

I AM grateful for knowing I've completely upgraded my epigenetic blueprint and kicked on my anti-aging and anti-disease genes in only seven days on a green juice fast.

I AM…

## Coming Homework:

Will you give yourself time to let your bowel digestion rest
—between 7 pm and 7 am or maybe fast one day a
week—even if one day includes skipping dinner one night
and no solid food until dinner the next day, green juicing or
water in between.

Will you open yourself to extending this into a 3-7 day fast?

Will you explore emotional eating and the emotions wanting
to be felt, healed and released?

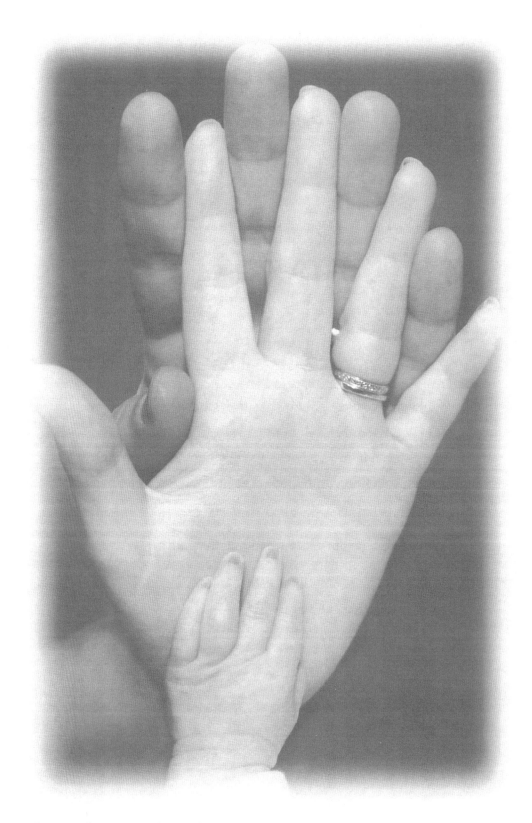

*Chapter 5:*

# *Connection, Mindbody Guidance, & Love*

"Too often we underestimate the power of a touch, a smile, a kind word, a listening ear, an honest compliment, or the smallest act of caring all of which have the potential to turn a life around." (Dr. Leo Buscaglia, 1972)

*When you have an expression that's coming from your heart, you'll always do the right thing... So watch that delicate balance between thinking too much and feeling things.*

*Brian Clement*

## *Being Seen*

Dr. Dean Ornish, physician and founder of Preventive Medicine Research, reminds us: "Loneliness is the number one contributing factor to illness." Seeking help and a healthy connection in community may be the difference between getting well or not. How and where we receive our guidance is significant and valuable, for it may determine whether we will flourish or wither.

Many of us began our lives in families that unconsciously felt more comfortable keeping us limited than helping us discover our very unique wide open, creative self, with accessibility towards our full potential.

Without judgement, we may acknowledge this as a large reclamation piece and move beyond the fear of being magnificent and of great value in a world desperately needing it. Misaligned eating is simply an old child imprint in the small emotional space of the brain and has primal fear of lack of food running the show. Yet, just step into nature, be still and feel the abundance!

Food is necessary fuel, such as oxygen. Seeing it as such, and choosing to run at our greatest capacity requires releasing our emotional attachments, finding the 'negative pair bonding,' and bringing compassionate inquiry into eating, while letting go of the rest. As Rameen Peyrow reminds us: we do not need to get rid of the addictive self, but simply bring awareness to it so we can refine self.

*The Hebrew root for spirituality means "breath, life." The word "counsel" means "guidance advisor" and "to keep one's wisdom." "To keep one's wisdom in every breath is a gift."*

*~ **Cyndi Doddick***

This reprogramming is done in sacred spaces of self inquiry through meditation, supported fasting, cleansing and re-inoculation; and through restoration of a leaky gut. This satsang is a coming home into a spiritual community of partnership, nature and beauty, access to enlightened teachers and functional medicine doctors; literature and prose music and chanting. It is a winding path of remembering the truth: **we are never alone and we are enough!** This can be messy, emotional and amazing!

I remember a time of extended isolation, in and out of hospital, and I remember surrendering to the thought: what if this is as good as it gets? I made my way to a yoga restorative class where the teacher played a cello piece called *The Poet*. I began moving in the deepest, rawest way. That one moment of the powerful cry of the cello marked the turning point of my health crisis. Grace is …sweet, sweet surrender!

*Oh My, the Healing Power in Surrendering to What Is Then*
*Letting It Go on the Next Breath!*

We are social by design. We align much more structurally stably with people who hold a higher vibratory energy. Just as when we put a log beside one that is already burning bright, we will catch on fire much more quickly. In the energy of using true divine guidance instead of force, we begin to understand that energy works like osmosis. If we are feeling misdirected or depleted, we are wise to entrain our minds into a higher frequency lifestyle that will allow our energy to flow freely, thereby nullifying illness. With this understanding we learn to expand, refine and re-refine the mind, the body, and the soul.

Spiritual guidance is the art of remembering our wisdom and breath. There is a Zen Buddhism-attributed saying that says, "how we do anything is how we do everything." This is the organic process of the unknown unity. Over time, as we heal our own hearts and heads, we become a more trustworthy friend and adviser, and we can also trust in sovereignty in which others are also finding their way home. As we begin to really trust our gut feeling and open to divine possibilities, healing may begin.

Meditation is essential in the process of learning when to seek counsel from the inner physician and when to let go …when to go beyond pharmaceutical solutions and study the methods that have healed many facing similar health challenges. Through meditation, we become aware much quicker when we are weaving into old patterns of codependency.

What is codependency exactly? It is a way of seeing the world that is often rooted in the misunderstanding we are responsible for another person's happiness. It has branches entwined into over-care taking, while being out of touch with one's own needs. It is a sure-fire way to have gut issues, for it is based in fear and survival. It was often founded in childhood when we developed negative reinforcement around being good or bad, and our intrinsic worth was connected to what we gave or did for others. Addressing this in counselling can be extremely helpful if we are to heal and navigate health.

Digestive disease expert, Jini Patel Thompson, who healed her own widespread Crohn's, and works with people with IBD through the protocol described in her book, *Listen to Your Gut: The Complete Natural Healing Program for IBS & IBD*, tells a story of a man with Crohn's, with whom she worked who refused to leave a family business he did not enjoy—even when the family dynamics, upon returning to work, contributed to rapidly increasing inflammatory markers. This is a story I hear over and over with people fearful of leaving people, places or things that have the potential to contribute to self-disconnect and flare-ups. (Anger turned inward, heating us up?)

> *If we can muster the strength to do what our gut is telling us,*
> *illness and our belly's messages can be the most amazing*
> *biofeedback therapy towards mindfulness.*

This has definitely been true for me as well—the incredible gift of my sensitive gut. Sometimes it is helpful to remember to let responsibility, respect, boundaries and grace weave their own webs of change. We witness patterns heal in ourselves over time and sometimes in just one sweet second of surrender, then we may settle down the nerve firing of the gut through the cultivation of both patience and gratitude. It is a miracle to feel gratitude for the simple things in: our breath, miraculous trees, new life, ability to change, and the awareness to know, in tough times, *"This too shall pass."* We may begin to see illness as the precious messenger it is.

The circles of infinite wisdom are renewing and reawakening through sacred sharing everywhere. Our life of paradox—we are much more ill as a society than ever before; and yet we are awakening.

Storytellers of natural laws and teachings, ancient microbial practices, earth keepers, peace-keepers, and integrative doctors are reigniting the Hippocratic Oath, (first do no harm). We have been given the plant-powered medicine and spiritual guidance for the healing of these times; plant medicine, regenerative soil, and farming practices, within beneficial bacteria.

Holistic guidance is fully integrated into eating, living and "being" in a way that moves us all towards awakening into a new upgraded normality to "awakened normality." In today's culture, the abnormal unhealthy has become normal.

In the light of knowing there are mossy microbial paths that lead us home to quietude and restful loving support, we can begin to explore how every choice affects our spirit, mindbody, and EarthGut, and our ability to be in healthy loving relationships with ourselves and others.

My work with wise teachers (both inner physicians and integrative teachers and physicians amongst the world), helped me understand that healing is much more probable when we call our energy and power back.

# *Authenticity & Coming Home*

Living a spiritual foundation and having a quiet mind requires time, space, and energy. In order for us to have love, meaning, and effectiveness, we must clear family patterns. This cannot be

*Deep listening to our beloveds is the greatest gifts we may bestow upon them.*

*~ Tami Hay*

stressed enough: without clearing our early theta-hypnotic imprints that do not lead us towards our divine spark of life, we could continue to relapse. This is assisted through finding and living peace. As adults, we can choose spiritual families that promote our well-being and anti-oppressive practices, within helpful supportive recovery groups and conscious living communities that require an honest self-inventory, healthy lifestyle changes and surrendering to a higher power for strength.

As we continue to develop our sacred relationship with the divine, we notice the divine everywhere—while layers of depth, caring, and compassionate guidance submerge into a safe harbour. For just beyond the veils of self-loathing habits is HEAVEN.

When our gut is suffering from dysbiosis, it is incredibly difficult to experience "heaven on earth." Many people's experience has been that, in times of acute inflammation, there is separation. Therefore, searching for the root cause to heal the inflammation may seem less motivating. Being in a supportive rejuvenation centre that individualizes our diet, with medical support and mindbody healing, was the biggest gift of self-love I gave myself.

People, sometimes, do not give themselves this gift because of the cost. For me, it would have been worth selling possessions and re-mortgaging a house, to deeply understand the root cause and answers to my healing. For in these centres, huge "mind-space" opened up the possibilities of "one disease and one cure." People arriving with cancer, diabetes, debilitating arthritis, and IBD were remarkably improved after only 21 days. The program included juicing, nutritional counselling, bodywork, and mindbody detoxification modalities.

This is the business of the "sacred relationship" (supporting our and each other's growth on all levels, including spiritual path), bringing truth and trust against the terror of disease. Terror may sound extreme, yet that is what many of us hold in our guts. In these precarious times, fear is everywhere.

**When we are truly listened to, the inner frightened and unprotected child may begin the process of trust.**

It is then that our live-food bowls and our bowels, brains, and healthy mircobes have a say in the matter; that our beauty, shining into God's will, will be made manifest. We gather …whole in hearts and community … stronger, and more humble and heart-centred.

*You come to me*
*Stories of yesteryear*
*Tattered yet never broken*
*Wise, seeker*
*Surrendering alas!*

*It is with great honour we sit at each other's table …*
*Us, both teacher and student*

*Humbled I am*
*That you have laid your vulnerability at my feet*

*I silently evoke a prayer*
*That I protect your heart, hold space for your soul*
*That I give you safe shelter*
*From your storm raging within*
*The organic process of healing begins*

*In our silent invocation of breath's gift*
*I hold the remembering*
*Regathering vessels of Divine sparks*

*Laughter and tears*
*Exhalation*
*Gathering*
*possibilities of liberation …*
*Returning …*
*Every breath a gift of remembering …*

# The Hero's Journey

This heroic journey into the unknown world of intimacy, vulnerability, and love's sweet mystery is not always comfortable. The root word of intimacy means "to know." Yet, the journey of the authentic self (beyond copying from old family dances) gives love a face, a name, and a purpose.

From boundary building to God-merging—far, far beyond ego gratification, we find balance and beauty, and we become present. This means letting go of our baggage, the goal-oriented anxieties of the future. The feminine flow is our way.

As a social work student many moons ago, I read Dorothy Briggs' *Three Hugs for Survival* and felt how few of us have ever had "genuine encounters" with grown ups—complete, undistracted human presence, which is critical for complete self-actualization.

**The heroic journey home is both a discipline and radical acceptance, as we consciously dance into reflecting God's consciousness in each other, then set up and invite in.**

"In order to be whole people, to do our work with integrity and honesty, we must show up with our whole selves, even those parts we do not like. If we can, we will discover something frightening, yet profound—that it is those parts we reject that make us good spiritual guides." (John Mabry, *Noticing the Divine: An Introduction to Interfaith Spiritual Guidance*, 2006)

Shamans remind us that our parents are only mortal beings. When we now source our energy from Mother Earth and Father Sky, we release drama infinity receptor sites and we are free to grow—UP! Not quite feeling that we belonged to our tribe is some of the inflammatory issues from childhood that sit in the belly and, when addressed and healed, can be a game-changer as in the vegan documentary *Game Changer*.

Maslow's hierarchy of needs, as seen through family dynamics, is often understood as engaging in searching for, denying, or permitting each other a specific "target goal" as we seek intimacy and nurturing. Many of us have been raised in families where our basic needs were not met. The base chakras, which are significantly affected in IBD, have often been placed in a hyper-survival mode, making it more difficult for people to access higher levels of intuition, such as what choices allow them to stay healthy. We are often working with the same shame that binds us.

Many of us have been raised with parents or community that were doing their best, yet were unable to hold our essence as a unique spark of divine—whether it was through food, lifestyle, or unhealthy social norms. These basic-root chakras, where digestive issues root deep, become the artful, continual creation of ancestral twine, unravellings toward whole-person healing. They release codependency that may lead us to make choices based on our inner child's need for acceptance, rather than grounded in right action for personal health, full empowerment, and healing. We see this continually in family gatherings surrounded by unhealthy food and drink expectations.

For myself and many others, this requires the courage and strength to seek out community that promotes wellness, personal truth, and conscious practices that support disease elimination. Space and boundaries were seldom respected in many families. When healing disease, it is of much value for us to redevelop our relationship with healthy sovereignty and beneficial boundaries on this space-and-time continuum. Many, many people are lonely. There is no motivation to heal if food that numbs us out is our only friend. Joining healthy community is key and life coaching is key; being seen is the balm!

A Sufi friend shares this in her practice, in which she is taught to ask herself four questions before speaking:

Is it true?
Is it kind?
Is it helpful?
Is it necessary?

These questions are amazing criteria for "conscious language" in the spirit of communication. Can we ask these questions inward first to understand if our self-talk is kind or not?

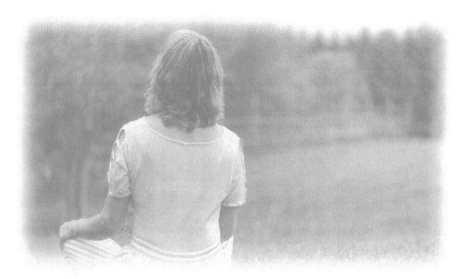

## Meditation:

As you bring your awareness to your breath here and now.

Explore your experience of your body.

Explore your breath and the sensations that occur and arise as you follow your breath into and through your body.

Explore what your tissues, organs and organ systems are communicating with you.

Explore the wisdom and guidance that your body shares with you moment-to-moment as you illuminate presence into each and every cell of your being.

What gift, wisdom, and guidance does your body have for you?

How does your soul want to live in this miraculous body you have?

Continue to follow your breath and continue to be curious and listen—in your own way to the unique way that your breath, body, and being want to communicate with you.

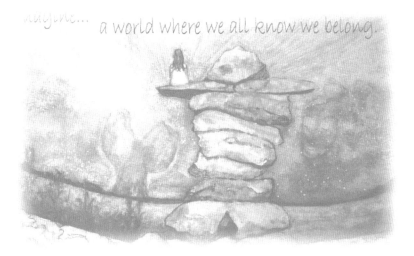

*imagine... a world where we all know we belong.*

## Gratitude:

I AM grateful for community and people where I'm able to be fully seen, challenged, and guided.

I AM grateful for a strong foundation towards peace and non-causal joy.

I AM grateful for my deepening connection to my inner wisdom through the clarity that my pure diet provides me.

I AM grateful for the infinite direction that is abundantly bestowed upon me in times of silence and stillness.

I AM grateful for following the guidance that has led me to the people, places, resources and food that bring me peace, health, and vitality.

I AM …

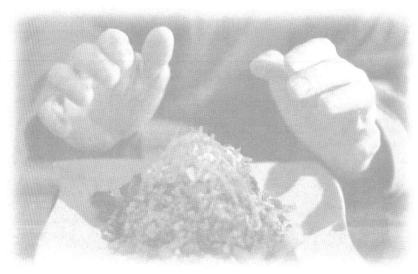

## Coming Homework:

Will you find a community of health seekers and conscious beings and connect regularly—share a meal, smile and share reciprocal loving-kindness?

Consider going to or receiving counsel from an integrative wellness centre to do a supported juice/water fast and or reset eating/lifestyle patterns.

Seek counsel and health-coaching support from beings you trust.

Trust and counsel yourself.

Get safe hugs and touch, transforming trauma to trust.

Pay it forward as you fill up with strength and hope.
We keep it by giving it away!

*The body resonates at the same frequency as
Mother Earth. So instead of only focusing on
trying to save the earth, which operates in
congruence to our vibrations, I think it is more
important to be one with each other. If you really
want to remedy the earth, we have to mend mankind.
And to unite mankind, we heal the Earth. That is the
only way. Mother Earth will exist with or without us.
Yet if she is sick, it is because mankind is sick
and separated. And if our vibrations are bad,
she reacts to it, as do all living creatures.*

**~ Suzy Kassem**

# Chapter 6:

# *Resonance, Addiction &*
# *Leaky Gut, The Great*
# *Peace Disrupter*

## *Leaky gut, Resonance the Great Peace Disruptor's*

I step into the smiles of my grandchildren's giggles and begin to remember the cellular resonance of love and joy. I remember that we come to this life with, and leave here, only love; and we spend all the time in between wanting to feel its freedom and peace once again. Addictions are born out of wanting relief, as are health crisis and kindness gatherings.

We resonate at the frequency of the level of our mindbody mineralization/ vitamin levels, hydration, ability towards

*Tight junctions are gatekeepers between the cells of your mega-membrane, which extend from the nasal cavity to the colon. Tight junction integrity can be impacted by environmental factors such as herbicides. As a result, your immune system can be overwhelmed.*

*~ Dr. Zach Bush*

detoxification; purpose/ability to serve; and our freedom from, what I refer to as intellectual obsessions.

There is a saying that originated from Alcoholic Anonymous that "wherever we go, there we are." Our resonant field attracts and repels the world in which we live. In this world, we do have some control in manifesting a life, we will feel at ease living in. What does all this have to do with mindbody EarthGut healing? Everything!

The gut—via food, drink, thoughts, bacteria, toxins, stress, harmony, and disharmony—is continually setting us up for either cravings or quietude. When we have intestinal hyper-permeability, we are continually leaking toxin back into our bloodstream. As we become more toxic, we often want food stuff that is less than healthy. For example, glyphosate in Roundup sprayed on conventional food has been proven to create dysbiosis hyper-permeability, otherwise known as leaky gut. Research suggests it can happen in as little as 12–16 minutes.

A healthy microbiome with diverse commensal microbes holds the integrity of the intestinal mucosa, preventing hyper-permeability of the mucosa integrity of the gut. Yet, pathogenic bacteria food such as gluten—which acts as a molecule-mimicker and produces zonulin, which increases intestinal permeability—and toxins such as glyphosate separate the healthy lining and create hyper-permeability—a leading precursor of most disease. I have never been able to remain in remission when I consumed even organic gluten!

The microbiome appears to be our epigenetic glue. It seems to come down to survival of the most adaptive microbes, the ones reestablishing their "gut instincts." This literally and emotionally may be what keeps us from coming unglued.

It was discovered that for every one neuron we have 7–9 microbes surrounding it and helping it do its work. The astrocytes and glial cells in the brain are found throughout the intestines! Yes, brain cells are in our bellies! In remembering the transference of these messengers through the vagus nerve, it would be wise to explore how everything that is happening in our gut directly is reflected in our brain, mindbody, intuition, connection, choices and emotional milieu.

**Other Hinderer's (Gut Busters):**

- Self-loathing and stress
- Antibiotics
- Gluten, (especially wheat dried by an application of glyphosate as a drying agent. just preharvested—yuk!)
  Gluten—as molecule-mimicker—invades and attacks thyroid (connection between thyroid and IBD)
- Alcohol
- Caesarean sections
- Sugar
- GMO and GE FOOD
- Endocrine disruptors and obesogens
- MSG
- Fructose
- Nicotine
- Lead
- Phthalates
- Bisphenols
- PBDE
- PFOA
- PCBs
- Dioxins

- Organophosphates
- Atrazine
- DDT
- Tributyltin
- DES
- Stress
- Radiation
- EMF

Our microbiota bacteria love community as well, and are constantly keeping the homeostasis of either pathogenic communities, such as mycotoxicity and Candida, or commensal bacteria communities grasping any bit of prebiotic and probiotics to return us back to health.

Resonant fields is why we hear the saying regarding neural pathways: "neurons that fire together, wire together." This is true for all three of our brains (head, heart, and gut), as well as gut-heart-mind. These hardwired habits are incredibly challenging to break—unless we rewire all three of our brains through detoxification, re-mineralization, re-inoculation and reconnection.

I gathered myself, through my much-needed time at wellness centres, where I was provided plenty of mindbody-soul food that allowed new pathways of possibilities to open me, truly saving my life. I rejuvenated my leaky gut with organic and biodynamic food, belly breathing, *ION\*Bione*, and EM-1 Probiotic. I gather myself daily on my yoga mat and in the forests. I remember I matter and that every choice I make, sets me free or traps me.

Yogic communities have often been a place to expand and realign, along with community who are focusing on whole-person healing to increase our 'vibe' so to speak.

Most research on addiction indicates that the "leakier" the gut, the more compulsive the behaviour. This is resonate energy fields upside-down. We crave "stuff" that keeps us at a certain vibration and emotional state that hard-wires and keeps feeding us what we are used to. This can be seen through the lens of resonance. We attract what we are roaming for and used to. If we really begin to understand that "what we are seeking is seeking us," as the great mystic poet Rumi tells us, then we may find a poetic way through this, with gentleness. Poetry, sound healing, and music helping us resonant at a frequency of deep listening, pure and living food the same.

This is where the crossroads meet—in this very moment when we bring deep listening to the equation. Remembering that we actually have a choice—to strengthen the groove of unhealthy habits or create ones that feed our precious-person health.

Through detoxification and re-inoculation of brain-supporting-microbes, we are continually resetting the nervous system, allowing new habits to rewire. The study of neuroplasticity is the understanding of the flexibility of our brain to be able to change at any age, strengthening new pathways which result in quickly achieving the results we are wiring towards; such as greater ability to think outside our unhealthy human norm.

Much precious prana is lost in the self-loathing of addiction. If you were to ask someone who gives power away to a substance or habit, they believe it all stems from a lack of willpower. The roots of addiction could have possibly begun in the absence of healthy guidance from people, microbes and nutrition from utero onward. No one is to blame here; just forward thinking, recreating and re-grooving toward healthy neural networks that set us up to be the "alkalarian alchemists" that has always been our birthright.

**It is critical information to know for healing, (abolishing guilt-invoking patterning), that addictions have never been "all in our head" or indicative of a weak will.**

What if, just for a moment, we imagine a universal resonance field within and outside our bodies—microbes, heart imprints, brain grooves deciding for us. What if what we resonate with is attracting people, places, and things that create peace, or no peace, from all the accumulation of what we have learned to be normal. What if normal no longer makes us happy, healthy, or holy? What if we can reset and strengthen new pathways faster than we thought, through a seven-day green juice fast, support and meditation?

As glyphosate has been known through science to create leaky gut, this is true also for most processed and additive foodstuff, alcohol, and many pharmaceuticals. Living nutrition helps us resonate at a frequency of deep listening and may be where the crossroads meet …in this very moment when we bring remembering and deep listening to the equation. Remembering what exactly?

**Remembering first and foremost that we actually have a choice; that we either strengthen the groove of old habit or create ones that feed health, liberation and purpose.**

- What if, just for a moment, we imagine a universal resonance field within and outside our bodies—microbes, heart imprints, brain grooves—deciding for us?

- What if we bring fierce compassionate inquiry into this space?

- What if what we "resonate" with is what we are attracting in people, places, and things that create peace?

- What if "normal" no longer makes us happy, healthy or holy?

What if we can reset and strengthen new pathways faster than we thought possible?

- Will a supported green juice or water fast support meditation?

Imagine… the permanent healing of the vulnerable coping strategies achieved in as little as three to ten weeks. Have hope, keep seeking, and persevere. Your being well matters.

Let us chant, tone, sing our way home, as we tonify our vagus nerve back into our heart into dominion over no other sentient beings, but rather reclamation over our birthright to be well, intelligent, and free!

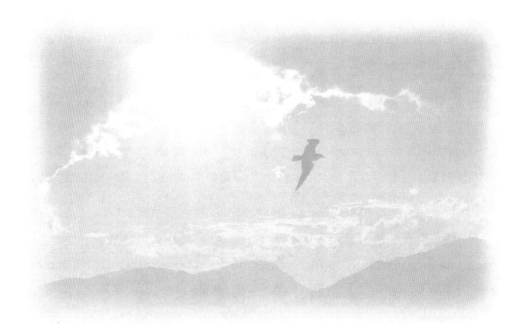

## Meditation:

Bring your full awareness to your in-and-out breath of your belly rising and falling. Feel the safety and spaciousness. Smile inward.

Keep belly breathing—letting thoughts and feelings arise and leave. Bring this to the next time you are grasping for love in an external substance, and see if your breath will ease the craving before you reach for the substance. Imagine yourself letting the thought form go … feel the spaciousness in that moment of non-reaction.

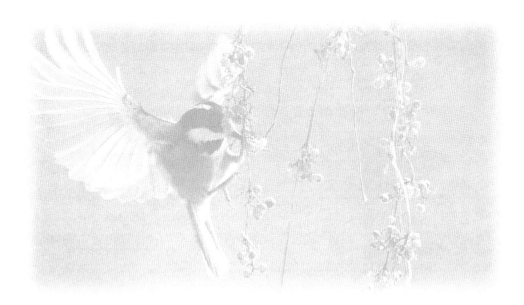

## Gratitude:

I AM free to choose life.

I AM free to feel and release.

I AM able to handle this without numbing out.

I AM…

## Coming Homework:

Will you begin to sing, dance, move, chant whole-healthy again, spending time outdoors in various ecosystems?

Will you breathe, drink water and find a healthy protein/fat; (ie. hemp heart) to fill the grasping when craving something that will not love you back?

Will you research gut bombs such as conventional and junk food, antibiotics, and stress, and release them?

Will you begin supplementations such as ION*Bione, Exalt and EM?

*When you open up your heart,*

*when you achieve a state of heart coherence,*

*the body manufactures 1300-1400 different*

*advantageous chemicals and hormones that*

*restore, regenerate, and strengthen the body's*

*immune system.*

*The body will naturally move*

*out of survival and diminish the stress*

*hormones so that it feels safe enough to create*

*(we cannot create in emergency mode).*

*As a result, your body will have more*

*energy for growth, repair, and healing.*

*Joe Dispenza*

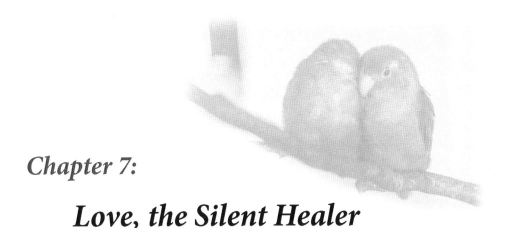

## *Chapter 7:*

# *Love, the Silent Healer*

### *Anti-inflammatory truth allows love accessibility.*

Love is not a concept. It is a living matrix that is deeper and older than our primordial need for food. For when infants are fed, yet not touched, they continually die of touch deprivation.

Love is who we are and maybe what keeps the stars, our spines, and our souls in alignment. Perhaps, just perhaps, when we see a forward-hunched older person, we may be seeing someone, for whatever reasons, who missed out on the love train and has spent their life lunging so far forward, when the present moment was not the loving, living matrix he needed to be here and now.

When we are privileged to be witness to a beautiful fresh love or a multi-decade loving kind one—love that is a conscious sacred union, this helps shift us back into conscious alignment. We are both participant and witness in love's sacred unions, a gift from beyond.

It is our birthright to live in love and freedom, yet so few of us know how to do this or have found communities that support such a life. We are taking the thousand-mile journey and practising presence while keeping our hearts wide open. For love is everywhere!

Feeling the love in beloved community soothes our senses and allows us to experience the love. It is impossible to heal without feeling loved and connected.

We can only heal when our heart is in it, when we bring energy to motion—emotion! What we are doing needs to matter in our heart of hearts or it will fizzle out quickly!

One morning, I watched while I lay under massive evergreens in this sacred mountain home. In the silence I was able to remember the beauty and effortless ease in both growth and grounding. In a world of sexual exploitation and pseudo-beauty attempts for love, it is essential we live in the power and essence of the following Navajo prayer:

## *Walk in the Beauty Way*

*In beauty all day long may I walk*
*Through the returning seasons, may I walk*
*On the trails marked with pollen, may I walk*
*With dew about my feet,*
*With beauty behind me,*
*With beauty below,*
*With beauty around me, may I walk*
*In old age wandering on a trail of beauty, lively, may I walk*
*In old age wandering, on trails of beauty, living again, may I walk*
*May my words always be beautiful*

When we look into the eyes of sacred love everywhere—in children, our beloved, and animals friends, we feel the beauty of a thousand hopes align. Alignment is love-aligning with truth, peace, and life times of tribal ancestral unwinding, calling us home.

Love is the gentlest brush of skin and the passing by of a smile, and the quiet homecoming of silence never so rich with unspoken words. Ahhhh, to be known! The ease and the caring and longing for the beloved to protect the open-hearted. Love whispers across the mountain peaks, shining down in pink and indigo, sunrise to sunset. Love comes without regret—alas!

## 11 Love Builders

1   Cultivate the art of self-love (for it is the only place where health-building choices will reside) by learning how to be well on this earth.

2.  Love others from the deep well of self-love, nurturing, and respect.

3.  Love the microbes that love you back.

4.  Live radical forgiveness.

5.  Allow yourself to be nurtured.

6.  Serve unconditional love.

7.  Speak from your heart.

8.  Listen, listen then listen some more, respecting sovereignty.

9.  Start every thought with kindness; kind words will follow.

10. Be true to your heart's dharma.

11. Choose a loving, conscious community.

# Love & Loving Connection Is Anti-Inflammatory

Oxytocin—the bonding hormone, has turned out to be anti-inflammatory. In a 2010 study, Gershon found: "Oxytocin levels can influence the digestive system as much as they influence the brain. Oxytocin has been proven to calm gastrointestinal inflammation, greatly reducing the risk of food sensitivities, autoimmune disorders and systemic infections."[21]

Stress is a prime driver in inflammation; love accomplishes the opposite. In an article by Donna Gates, author and teacher of *The Body Ecology Diet and Is Your Stress Causing Leaky Gut and Candida?*, she shares research on how stress creates brain fog by creating intestinal permeability. The release of cortisol and nor-epinephrine shuts down digestion and bacteria polymorph to unhealthy bacteria. It is challenging to feel love when we are severely inflamed.[20]

I felt this intimately eight months after my son died. My heart starting beating an abnormal beat after every normal one. I saw a cardiologist, knowing it would correct itself as my broken heart healed. This proved true. The cardiologist tells me he sees this correction with "heart healing" over and over again.

In a University of Zurich study, oxytocin was found to lower the stress hormone cortisol. This was shown in loving daydreams and hugging someone, whom you love.

In an article by Dr. Bill Miller, I love you... Actually I love your Microbiome, he links fascinating research regarding our partner choices and their microbiome. It turns out our choice in partners is based on an innate survival defence: we choose partners with microbes capable of healthy mating. Much of this information is exchanged in kissing, through the microbiota on the back of the tongue. Kissing reduces stress, as does cuddling together, holding hands, tea breaks. [21]

### *Three hugs a day for survival, even if you are hugging yourself*

*Can you sit with me?*
*Really sit, quiet and still*
*In the centre of the fire*

*The vulnerable and messy*
*The forgiveness and the love*
*Unprotected and vast*
*In the emptying of clutter*

*Can you sit with me here?*
*Can you hear my silence*
*Feel my heart*
*As I yours*
*And not jump into something more familiar-chatter and clutter*

*Can you lay with me*
*Breathe my every space, unknown still to me?*
*Can we hold each other to the fire, to our hearts?'*
*And never shrink back*
*Can we just be?*
*Heartbeat and breath*
*Our only compass*

When we talk about cohesion, interconnection, and our second brain—the heart—we would be wise to connect with the *Heart Math Institute*. Since 1990, they have been conducting extensive research on the mindbody-heart connection. They have helped us understand how the heart is our compass in life. The more we explore the depth of our hearts, the less we can deny the power of our interconnection and the heart, as our central communicator for our entire body and our navigator into wiser and more heart-centred choices.

## *The Heart-Mind Microbiome*

Dr. David McClelland at Boston University defines love as a body/mind state that includes the entire human system, immune system, and heart. Since our greatest immunity is in our microbiome system, then stress-free, bonded, loving relationships are literally good for our gut. McClelland also showed a remarkable difference between lovers who exerted power as opposed to the strengthened immune systems of lovers who deeply understood the power of love. When we learn to tap into our hearts' healing, we not only prolong our lives, but the lives of all the heart-centred souls around us. Perhaps we should heed the words of Pearsall, "The most important health warning of all is to 'have a heart.' "[22]

Twenty-one days after conception, the muscle of our heart, with over two billion muscle cells and 40,000 neurons, begins instantly to pump signals to both our gut and our brain.

The heart-mind interacts both electrically, via the vagus and spinal nerves, and chemically through the endocrine system. These heart neurons are in continual connection with the brain/microbiome and it is now understood that the brain obeys bacteria [23]

The heart as an endocrine gland releases peptides and hormones, such as oxytocin, and allows bonding to occur that might otherwise be difficult. It is now better understood that the inability to connect and bond may be more rooted in the bacteria, as oxytocin pathways may be interrupted when *Lactobacilli* strains are absent. How much of a role does our microbiome play into our ability to live with a connected heart?

## STORY:

This story is from The Heart's Code. It is one of those stories that touch deeply and you long to share it. It is about a boy who received a new heart and started calling his dog by a different name. The mystery was solved when his parents met the donor's parents and learned the different name was the name of the deceased boy's dog.

Our olfactory, like most of our ancient cellular memory, is deeply encoded in the heart. This may be why it is dangerous for us to live with someone constantly cooking fresh bread if we have chosen for our health to release gluten. I wish to add a little introduction from the HeartMath Institute book, *The Science of the Heart*, for every word sums up our beautiful interconnection.

## HeartMath Institute is valuable beyond belief in why we keep our hearts open, as in this quote:

"Early on in our research we asked, amongst other questions, why people experience the feeling or sensation of love and other regenerative emotions as well as heartache in the physical area of the heart. In the early 1990s, we were among the first to conduct research that not only looked at how stressful emotions affect the activity in the autonomic nervous system (ANS) and the hormonal and **immune systems**, but also at the effects of emotions such as appreciation, compassion and care. Over the years, we have conducted many studies that have utilized many different physiological measures such as EEG (brain waves), SCL (skin conductance), EKG (heart), BP (blood pressure) and hormone levels, etc. Consistently, however, it was heart rate variability, or heart rhythms that stood out as the most dynamic and reflective indicator of one's emotional states and, therefore, current stress and cognitive processes. It became clear that stressful or depleting emotions such as frustration and overwhelm lead to increased disorder in the higher-level brain centres and ANS and which are reflected in the heart rhythms and adversely affects the functioning of virtually all bodily systems. This eventually led to a much deeper understanding of the neural and other communication pathways between the heart and brain. These influences affect brain function and most of the body's major organs and play an important role in mental and emotional experience and the quality of our lives."[24]

The heart rules so much of our biology and many of our decisions about whether or not we can heal or whether we are even worthy enough. The heart appears to directly interact with our gut and signalling. The above excerpt is incredibly valuable in understanding the heart's role in healing.

Dr. Paul Pearsall, author of The Heart's Code, has studied psychoneuroimmunology and has discovered, when working with heart patients, the number one factor on how rapidly they heal or the severity of their condition was how deep their heart-centred connections were in family and community. Dr. Pearsall calls this "L" energy:

"I have been using the letter 'L' to represent the vital life force that may come from and is circulated by the heart. We have reported data that indicates that two persons in a loving bond working on the same experiment together do not simply combine what our staff calls 'individual subtle energy signals.' Instead, there seems to be a coupled subtle energy effect that is a unique blend of each other's energy foot signature."[25]

Yet preventable heart disease is the leading cause of death. Dr. Esselstyn, a cardiologist surgeon has proven thousands of times over that a whole-food, plant-based diet reduces heart disease, (as many others in the Physicians' Committee for a Responsible Medicine).[2]

We know our conventional food is creating systemic inflammation and inflaming our hearts. I am also aware, in times of quietude, the karmic connection in no longer partaking in the inhumane way animals are treated for our entertainment and food. Do we eat their broken-hearted, pained bodies with reciprocal diseased and unsettled effects?

# A Grateful Heart to Reduce Inflammation

I'm curious about the ripple effect of including another person in the gratitude circle through deep appreciation. We are seeing these infinite love and gratitude circles everywhere. The amplification of positive love and energy in a space and the "one energy field" resonance of people coming together for peace cannot be overlooked.

Cultivating gratitude in the very moment relaxes the body instantly; such as:

## Meditation:

As we take the focus off of what is frustrating us and put it on breathe in and breathe out, we can cultivate gratitude for: the sun's warmth and light; the trees for their incredible oxygen and beauty; the divine for the infinite energy; the microbial-rich earth for her constant forgiveness and constant regeneration, and the other souls in meditation or savasana sharing their light with us.

## Prayer:

It is recommended that before we ask God for what we want, we should thank God for what we have.

## Gratitude Journal:

Keep a gratitude journal. Writing down five things you are grateful for each morning and evening is often life-changing and reduces much stress.

## Count Our Blessings:

This is an opportunity to look at the possibility that all that happens in God's world has the potential to be for our good. It's a huge possibility to swallow and digest (pun intended) when we are not feeling well, but sometimes contemplating how dis-ease can slow us down enough to look at what is really going on and accessing the physician within, could be worth its weight in gold. People from some of the most financially challenged countries smile the most.

## Smile:

Dr. Aung, a qigong master and TCM doctor from my neck of the woods, emanates love from every cell of his being as he tells us smiling and the qigong practice of smiling into our organs has a profound effect on our happiness and well-being. There was an amazing UC Berkeley study that took a large group of clinically depressed individuals, put them in front of a mirror daily for 20 days and they had to smile deeply at themselves for 20 minutes. Depression alleviated in all of them.

## Verbally and Mentally Thanking People:

If we really want the last word, let it be "thank you." Stopping ourselves in the middle of a slippery slope of frustration and the need to be right; and coming back into our space of divine breath and non-codependency, we should close our eyes, if even for a minute, and give thanks.

One of these practices that I have found valuable is this loving-kindness Buddhist prayer:

**May you be filled with loving-kindness**
**May you be well**
**May you be peaceful and at ease**
**May you be happy**

I like to use this prayer in present, already so tense …you are filled …

We direct this prayer inward first, repeating three times or more; first cultivating love for self, then directing it outward towards cultivating love towards another. It helps us connect to the basic needs of all humans.

*STORY:*

Mentoring a young man with CD, who was trying to decide on whether to begin a strong immunosuppressant medication on day four of a juice/water fast. After 3–4 days of green juice bowel resting, his abdominal pain significantly subsided. He was very concerned about what would happen when he started introducing solid food back into his diet. He spoke of the stress and emotional turmoil that had plagued him in his eight years with CD. I had just arrived home from a beautiful yoga practice, feeling light and grateful, as I usually feel when connecting breath and body with other yogis for 90 minutes.

I shared with him how absolutely grateful I am for the lessons and upgrades I have received in the open and ever-changing emotion towards making peace with myself hence Crohn's disease. He looked at me extremely puzzled, as if to say "the gut-brain axis must have played a number on you during your inflammatory years." It did not seem like a logical way to think about such a debilitating disease. Yet I am just one of many who has transformed through the lens of dis-ease. Many people have been able to access the incredible gift of self-actualization when curing what is so-called incurable, and go on to live a richer, more purposeful, and inclusive lovelife.

## *Love Is Everywhere: A Love Story*

Here, now, sharing time with a friend in the solitude of a country lake home. She is attending to the dark night of the soul and emerging a butterfly even if she has not felt all of her metamorphose yet. But I see it, as a witness and a friend, for I have walked a thousand miles in her moccasins. The Trojan Horse that led me through the dark forest into the shimmering green emerald woods came with a different name. Mine UC and CD, and hers cancer, yet the transformation and letting go remains the same. We both needed to shed the layer of illness illusion to feel the illumination that love is everywhere!

Her question to me, "Why is it that so many people don't love themselves?" She has become deeply involved in a sacred and conscious church called *The Center for Spiritual Living* and is healing every limited belief that has constantly plagued her beautiful body and soul. The theme, so common to many yet spoke by few: "you are not okay, you do not belong, you are alone." "Absolutely everyone," she says,"only wants to feel loved. Love is everywhere and yet a lot of times I still feel like a monster. I never was supposed to be here. How can anybody survive or thrive when we are thought of like that?"

# *I Remember that Metamorphous:*

In my last hospitalization with CD, my daughter found me on the bathroom floor saying: "Mom, you have to go to the hospital." Worry in her beautiful eyes. I had been sitting on the toilet trying to pass anything— except my bowels were almost swollen shut with inflammation. Even passing mucus and blood sent so much pain riveting through my body that I would almost pass out or vomit, or both. The last thing I remember was coming to this place far away from the pain-body I felt on the bathroom floor. I felt warm intense peace and light and immense love—it was beyond. I wanted so much to stay. But something, I do not know what, put me back in my body. For how long this occurred, I cannot say— minutes? All I know for certain is I felt different, lighter one hour later in that hospital bed, IV drip for hydration. There I was in a room with an older woman under close medical care and something felt very different this hospitalization. Fear had left me, despair was gone and deep sadness released. I was still in the same weak, grey-skinned, fragile body—yet my eyes were brightening. I was able to get a glimpse of that little girl who loved to catch frogs, eat violets and clover, and sing songs at Sunday school.

So when the woman next to me, amputated, catheterized and seeping with sores from a life riddled with self-loathing, loneliness and diabetes reached out, divine love answered. It was in that moment I remembered what I felt on the bathroom floor: "You will go back to help people remember that they are loved, lovable AND they do belong!" She asked me what I did for work. Massage therapy and energy work, I responded. "The only time I get touched," she said, "is when I receive medical care. It has been so long since I have had a massage."

There I was, IV pole in hand, holding on to furniture to get myself to her bed. I sat next to her. Head resting on her bed to conserve the little strength I had, I held her hand with my close IV hand and touched her heart with the other. I felt grace flood in—it may seem unhealthy, me comforting her at this time in my health, yet it was action without thought, action from somewhere beyond. This is the greatest connection that heals. Illness can be an amazing awakening!

That next eight days in the hospital were significantly different—I joked with the doctors, assured my family I was okay, painted trees and water, and devoured Louise Hay's book, *You Can Heal Your Life*. I transitioned easily into a mindset of awakening into a world of affirmative mantras.

I told my daughters I would never be in the hospital for CD again.

That was thirteen years ago and I have felt deep purpose and a steeped sense of gratitude every day since; not every second of every day, yet each day.

This is often the re-collection of change felt by people close to the veil and near-death returners. I told my friend this story on a spring snowstorm morning as we watch siskins fly from the pussy willows to the full feeder, happy-free. There is so much more than this mindbody!

*Why do so many of us not feel the love when love is everywhere?*
*Are we longing for our connection of missing microbes and "L" energetics?*

*I believe most of us don't have community, proper nutrition, genuine connection, parents with a template of unreasonable happiness, uncensored joy, or roots in divine purpose and spiritual nutrition.*

It is predicted by shamans, medicine people—enlightened beings everywhere—that this very time on the planet, we will experience an elevation of conscious being that we have never seen before, and staying unconscious would become considerably difficult. We have suffered and we can turn that into deep compassion when we heal our spirit and know we are only here for love. It is up to us. Healer, heal thyself …for by doing so, we help heal the next seven generations unseen.

In *The Course of Miracles*, a miracle is described as a shift in perception. In these precarious times, huge shifts in perception are happening with people everywhere. My friend and I embrace, smudge sage and pray. In a world of isolation, sadness, and disconnect, spiritual counselling can offer a refuge and return harmony, allowing people to feel the love energy that is paramount for healing. Some shamans tell us we are too toxic to journey our way home, too deficient of a body-electric to remember. Antidote: Earth Mother, veganic/organic food, soil, and lots of love.

## Meditation:

Find a quiet place to close your eyes and breathe.

As the rhythm of your breath softens and relaxes you, see yourself disconnecting with the thought forms that are associated with the stress of dis-ease. They lift away.

See every thought released onto a prayer to a God of your understanding and later onto a paper.

When you are ready, you can write, from this place, all the past that contributes to stress and disease.

Find a place to give this paper gift to the fire; you can wrap it with a flower, some sage or any other offering. When you release it to the fire, turn your back and allow the ashes behind you and your past to no longer take energy up in your precious energetic existence.

Allow yourself to be still, feeling the support of Mother Earth beneath you. Feel yourself as a piece/peace of both Heaven and Earth. Sink deeper and deeper still. Breathe into your heart and feel it expand and soften.

Feel yourself through the heart pulse of the earth; feel hope is reachable as long as your heart is beating.

Smile into your heart. Think of someone you love deeply and feel how that softens you.

Rewrite your life without limit. Create from this place!

## Gratitude:

I AM supposed to be here, for my heart's still beating.

I AM resilient and open.

I AM open to love and discern what creates chaos and give it to the fire under the new and full moons.

I AM well.

I AM grateful for all the resources I have that allows me to release the stress of inflammation throughout my mindbody.

I AM grateful for the ability now to slow down and listen to the messages this dis-ease is teaching me or to move when my body is asking.

I AM grateful for how quickly my body responds to relaxation and quietude.

I AM…

## Coming Homework:

Journal and list life-giving loves in your life daily. Gratitude journals change lives! Keep a gratitude journal beside your bed and write 3–5 things in which you are grateful for, each morning and night.

In your release journal, write old thought forms, that no longer serve, bringing to the fire all that no longer shines. This is great to perform on new moons.

By burning these past teachings with gratitude for the learning, you are making space for health and new energy and life force to return. Turning your back as they burn is a symbol of turning away from the past and going forward!

Breathe deeply, softening and opening your heart daily, saying, "I am safe! I am loved! I am enough!"

"Now, knowing better, we can act better,
we can live better, and give the animals,
our children and ourselves a
true reason for hope and celebration.


There is no way to overstate
the magnitude of the collective spiritual
transformation that will occur when
we shift from food of violent oppression to
food of gentleness and compassion."

~ Dr. Will Tuttle [75]

Miracles do not happen to you?
Yet Precious, here you are!
A belly born of a universe
Maybe a million years ago?

A bite of this sweet biome
To change your cells today
A garden feast of rainbow cuisine
To light your microbes array

A star is born and a star goes out
And all you love and despise
Will be a distant molecule
Disguised before your eyes!

You think of me and I think of you
At that very same momento
Quantum leaps across the world
Entanglement the 'vibe'

And every crevice of our skin
Is yours just for this time
How could we even conceive of 'self'
Your eyes once maybe mine

Each breath in and each breath out
Our molecules drift over there
How could we ever feel alone
Our biome we ALL share!

# Chapter 8:

# *Loving our Anatomy, Digestion, & Physiology:*

## *Energetic and Physical Anatomy and Physiology*

"I believe in the circuit of the stars in times like these, and its magnetic properties, the human beings!" Xavier Rudd

All of our organs, when given the right environment of mindbody, have the ability to heal. This is an absolute truth, not often spoken of in symptom-suppression and dis-ease management models of 'sick-care'. We are prana, life force and ever-changing tissue. We need our energy to repair, rebuild, and be joyful. Your mindbody interacts each and every second.

This primordial truth of our oneness sits in our first root, chakra, and when integrated it may send messages through the Kundalini river (our spine is often referred to as our Kundalini river of light in energy medicine), from earth's roots through to the beyond.

We are all magnetically connected—every microbe, every cell, nerve, fibre, organ, gland, bone, muscle, lymphatic tissue, blood and cardiac-energetic heart. In the realm of anatomy and physiology, many of us have been educated to view our incredibly interconnected bodies as organs that function separately from one another, separate from our biome. Yet, this cannot possibly be true! Much research reveals the study of interconnection; they are all connected through microbial mystery.

From a systems perspective, the human organism is a truly vast, multidimensional information network. It may consist of many subsystems, but they are all intrinsically interwoven through the matrix of the one field connecting intimately with our microbiome: up to 99% of each of us is not human bacteria, but rather dust of the earth.

When we open our spiritual hearts, we encode into the one matrix of the universal heart. In this place, we find peace and coherent wisdom, allowing us to hear the eternal music of connection. Here we abandon inharmonious thought, desire, and habit. In light of our beautiful interwoven self, it may be of benefit to explore all of the following as one system: esoteric energy, acupuncture meridians, anatomy and physiology—all focusing deeper into understanding how each action brings us either into health or further away.

It is simple to see how a person lives and thinks by watching their physiology.

Sadness, for example, becomes our structured physiology quickly—hunched shoulders (heart protection), downward gaze, etc. Twelve-step groups often use the phrase, "fake it until you make it." Joe Dispenza may refer to this as deep visualization focus until our physical correlates to what our deeply-focused mind created. We return to perfect health much quicker when we live with hope and living "as if it were so" …live, speak, and position our anatomy in such a way that suggests we are already aligning into health in this very moment. This may be very difficult for people who suffer from dysbiosis of the microbiota, yet still possible.

The connection of the gut to the brain through the vagus nerve and the microbiome are deeply researched topics in science today. But the interface of the brain/gut barrier is often overlooked in modern medicine, overlooked in many brain/gut disorders—from degenerative disease to inflammatory bowel disease depression right through to autism. The work of Dr. Perlmutter, a trailblazing neurologist, speaks volumes about the interconnection of all systems and how it relates to the microbiome.

## *We Must Be Connected, Hydrated, Mineralized & Alkalized to Be Well & Experience Joy*

Enzymes are essential to life. They are the great transformers of every hormone, vitamin, mineral, fat, protein tissue, and carbohydrate. It's becoming very clear from the multitude of research and books written over the last couple of years that enzymes, hydration and mineral/vitamin synthesis are essential to gut health and our mental/emotional well-being.

## *Hydration for Life*

We can HEAL when we infuse and connect with our cleansing and sacred element, water. A friend of mine from the Cree Nation said his grandfather told him when he was a wee lad, "One day, boy, we will have to buy our water." My friend found this statement incomprehensible, yet here we are.

Water's main function is to bring life into the cells, to literally light us up! Water transports information, it has memory. This has been known for a long time. It either has the memory of structure and minerals, hydrating us cellularly or is mediocre at best in helping us fully.

Myths: clear pee equals enough water and we all get thirsty. When we have clear pee this simply means water is not reaching our cells. By the time we become thirsty we are already dehydrated, eventually in extreme dehydration, (as seen in many young and old), we may lose our thirst signalling mechanism. Anything we ignore long enough, will stop trying to get our attention. This is dangerous, as our incredible biology is shutting down the alert signalling, which is paramount for our health.

## Hmmm, What Is WATER Exactly?

Water is us, earth, life. Water is much more than two hydrogen atoms and one oxygen atom, creating a dipole, which allows water molecules to connect to each other through the hydrogen bond. Hydrogen means donating electrons, therefore water is incredibly dynamic in nature, exchanging one of two hydrogens with electron energy. This process is known as hydrolysis and has a life-giving effect on the mindbody. Therefore, water is also responsible for ATP synthesis utilizing energy. Minerals in water are known as ions—the more minerals we have, the greater chance cellular hydration is occurring with intake of water. The perfectly structure water in fruit and vegetables, in their organic raw living state, hydrates us with the memory of pure structured water, as vegetables and fruit are mostly water.

In the book, *Your Body's Many Cries for Water*, Dr Fereydoon Batmanghelidj talks about dehydration equalling inflammation and water essential in turning off histamine. The main function of histamine in the body is water regulation. Most inflammatory issues such as colitis, dyspepsia, rheumatoid pain (water is needed to lubricate the joints), back pain, (specifically low back pain and sciatica) are chronic symptoms of dehydration. Dehydration causes: acidity, toxemia, accelerates aging, and damages DNA which decreases the flow of hydrogen into the cells.[26]

Dehydration has been known to create every issue: emotional and mental disturbances, osteoporosis, constipation, headaches, fatigue (especially daytime and morning fatigue), because we are incredibly dehydrated in the morning. Be the STUDY OF ONE and start drinking electron donating-electrolyte water and eating biodynamic fresh food! Our mitochondria, the energy powerhouses of our cells, can not make ATP without proper hydration. Live food in its "unbroken wholeness" and structured water delivers to the cells well! The most basic reason for all disease and illness is cellular dehydration.

Every biochemical reaction in the body requires water hydration. The water in live organic vegetables is structured and mineralized. Many of us often realize how much more hydrated we are when drinking raw green juice intermittently with water or electrolytes, than water alone. The human body is two-thirds water, the blood 80% water, the brain 80% water, (same sweet water content as trees).

## pH Balance & Our Body Electric

We are biochemical individuals, with control over our ever-changing inner ecosystem. An alkalized, hydrated life is a culture of self-love made manifest. This is a culture of living waters, live mineralized sun food and a universal breath pulsating from the core of Pachamama, whispering the remembrance of our non-dualistic connection.

An alkalized electron donating body is a body with a pH of 7.4. The p stands for "protenz," from the Latin word for potential. The H stands for hydrogen.

Alkaline water is (OH-) and is capable of generating a high-voltage body. Alkalinity is energizing, magical and invites cool, calm, collected, and creative people who understand purpose. The pH has only to drop to 6.9 before a person's brain begins to get hazy. Perfect homeostasis helps eliminate cancer, viral/bacterial infections, arthritis, etc., as all of these imbalances need an acidic environment to survive. Some of the minerals that provide healing frequencies are: iridium, iodine, calcium, magnesium, sodium, sulphur, phosphorus, silicon, chlorine, and oxygen.

In acidic systems, water cannot electrically interface with cells. The pH balance of alkalinity is the most significant requirement for cellular hydration for our mind and body. There is not one part of the body's system that can function in the absence of electrically charged, available water. The frequency of the mindbody increases or decreases depending on hydration at the cellular level.

Water's role is to act as a transporter of electrons. Water has a subtle adhesive quality in bonding cell membrane structures. It acts as an antioxidant. High-electron water neutralizes free radicals. Our body is the body electric. Every transfer of electrical energy requires minerals. Blessing our earth, water and food may increase the absorption of nutrients many fold. This was the study in the book *Messages From Water*.

Let us choose to consciously rehydrate, reawakening our connection to our EarthGut, our sacred mineralized matrix and the hows and wheres to source our real medicine. Minerals for deep, cellular hydration are grown in mineral and bacteria-rich soils, eaten uncensored and live from soil rich in microorganisms. Every healthy body can be traced back to having sufficient minerals. We must be healthy to feel good.

*Hydration and water are our 1st protocol for detoxification!*
*No hydration, no healing, no health!*

There is not one sick person who is cellularly hydrated! Yet our system is set up for dehydration: science has proven EMF exposure dehydrates our system; toxins in food and water; stress in all its forms are extremely dehydrated. How is your society dealing with stress? Often people are numbing out with fast food, alcohol, media, all of which are further dehydrating the system. The key to hydration is the ability for the water to cross the membrane into the cell's mitochondria. This requires electron energy—this requires health.

In order to be of love and service, remembering who we are, we must be super-hydrated—mineralized, structured, electrolyte beings.

*If the mitochondria hold more light than the sun, how can we even conceive of a single lonely self, fumbling through a disease-controlled world?*

How can we not want to light up those inner cellular mitochondria with water and more mineralized water!!

For the cellular self to become fully hydrated, it may take months. Yet, the body is incredibly self-healing by design. It is a process worthy of attention; eating fibre-rich food assists in the body's ability to hold onto water as does a diet rich in water-soluble vegetables and fruit.

In this summary from Dr. Zach Bush, we begin to understand the gift of water:

> "Water is the ultimate in the scrubber system, so water is really the ultimate mechanism by which we get toxins out of our body, by which we clear the natural exhaust waste and break down products. Oxidants need to be cleaned out of the system and nothing on earth scrubs as well as water does. There's so much confusion with respect to simply drinking water as being the solution; yet, if not properly balanced, will actually cause you to urinate that water out really quickly and not get it inside the cell.

The clinical manifestation of aging and inflammation is ultimately one of a loss of fuel production at the mitochondrial level as you get dehydrated. As you fail to get oxygen and hydrogen in the form of water inside the cell you lose the ability for those mitochondria to be cranking out all of that energy that is not just a muscle energy. This is actually the energy that is used for cellular repair replacement and the whole anti-aging effort. You can't talk about mitochondrial health or mitochondrial fuel production without talking about water. Those two are absolutely inseparable."

# Minerals Essential for Hydration we are Usually Deficient in:

## Potassium

Most people don't get enough. The average intake is only half as much as sodium. A healthful intake is five times more potassium, than sodium, which is easily gotten by eating a more organic vegetable / fruit-based diet.

## Chloride

The synergist to both sodium (NaCl) and potassium (KCl), it is essential to keep these items in proper balance.

## Calcium

This mineral is essential for proper cardiac and muscle function; if too low one can get muscle cramps along with poor sleep and irritability.

## Magnesium

When low muscle spasms can occur. This mineral is also crucial for maintaining a healthy airflow and to help keep blood pressure balanced. Crave chocolate? Probably magnesium deficient.

## Trace Minerals - The Forgotten Minerals

Our cells cannot make adenosine triphosphate (ATP), which stores the energy we need to do just about everything we do, without proper hydration. Live food in its unbroken wholeness and structured water deliver!

# Very Basic Digestion Physiology

Our miraculous and ever-changing anatomy and physiology stores every memory, every belief, and every pattern within the "issues in our tissues." Muscle and tissue have memory. When the body is not working well, it simply means there is congestion in our system we must clear out.

In studying our physical form, we may see the unseen in the way we stand, walk and talk: from shoulders hunched and tired, we see years of a heavy-hearted mind turned into a structure of a tired anatomy. A straight, flexible and free gait may indicate a person who is resilient and able to move through life with flow and ease, letting go of the past or fear of the future.

We have an energetic body. In yoga, this anatomy is known as koshas, chakras, and nadis; to name but a few. In Western medicine, we focus on the study of flesh, bones, muscles, tissue and organs. When we become participants of commitment to self-inquiry, we may breathe into these congested areas and bring spaciousness to them. In wonder, we may begin to understand the choices we make and how they are affecting our health;

for example:

"Gluten gives me cold sores or cankers and I feel down when I eat it, meat makes me tired and anxious, I overeat when I feel lonely to stuff this emotion down." etc.

When Hippocrates said, "death lurks in the intestines—bad digestion is the root of all evil," he was planting the seed to begin our understanding of energy and plant medicine, and helping us make the connection—our intestines and digestive system communicate intimately with our brain. Now science is looking through the lenses of the microbiome, along with the vagal nerve connection, in gut-brain wellness.

Some may say the microbiome is the third brain, after the heart, due to the heart's intricate ability to store memory and life-force information. Neuropeptides are found throughout the intestinal lining—a gut reaction or sore tummy is a brain message.[27]

## *The Digestive Microbiome Tube*

The digestive tract is 10–15-feet long from nasal/mouth to anus. This single-cell, mucosa lining is perfectly designed to protect, break down, digest food, absorb, and assimilate nutrients, eliminate waste, and breed intestinal flora. A running nose, sinus issues, and lung disorders have been known to be soothed and relieved through bowel cleansing.

The folds and sub-folds of the intestinal walls are filled with villi and micro-villi, increasing the contact area two hundred fold, an absorption haven. Both mechanical chewing (complete mastication of food essential for digestive health) and digestive enzyme secretion; along with satellite organs such as salivary glands, liver, gallbladder, and pancreas, work together interchangeably. One day of not eliminating fully and these bowel toxins back up into liver.

Unconscious haphazard eating and poor food-combining, promotes putrefaction which result in toxic byproducts; bowel irritation and inflammation throughout the digestive system. This is why fasting works so well; it gives the digestion a chance to catch up with elimination and clears congestion in digestive organs so dis-ease has no place to breed.

Hence, mindful mastication of our food, while connecting with all aspects of the energy of healthful food, is paramount. It adds greater symbiosis by tuning in, with a felt sense, to the trees and earth from which it was grown, to the growers and cuisine food artists, to the Creator, and to the gift of health we are giving ourselves and the planet by eating this way.

Food digests easily when we are in a parasympathetic state; cool, calm and reconnected versus a sympathetic state of stress. It is best not to eat when not feeling calm and wait to make eating a meditative experience, a gift to give oneself.

## *The GALT*

When foreign materials and toxic undigested matter get through, the gut associated lymphatic tissue (GALT), which is the warehouse for 80% of the body's defence and life-saving lymphatic tissue and bacteria, begins its action-packed job of keeping us protected. When we keep the GALT on hyper mode, by constantly ingesting allergens or hard to digest non-food stuff, we rob nerve energy out of our system, and we become enervated-- unable to produce enough power to keep us detoxified.

When this thin velcro of our single-cell bowel lining is exposed to glyphosate, pesticides and allergens, zonulin- (the protein that releases the signal to open up the tight junctions to release larger toxic particles, then close tight again), stays on overdrive. We develop intestinal hyper-permeability, "leaky gut," allowing toxics to roam freely throughout the bloodstream- even crossing the blood / brain barrier. This is a health crisis!

The giant crypts that line our intestinal wall (unfolded would cover a football field), are a perfect breeding ground to resident microorganisms —bacteria heaven. There are hundreds of different good bacteria which can weigh as much as the three pound liver—all working with the immune system to fight invaders.

The intestinal wall has a layer of connective tissue, which holds in place the blood vessels and collects what is absorbed. Another concentric layer is the muscle cells, squeezing the digestive tract forward. In between is a discontinuous layer of immune system cells and a multitude of bacteria. Tiny nerve fibres touch the intestinal walls of the digestive tract, directing and regulating functions such as peristalsis. Contraction, timing and, strength of this action is all governed by the nerve filaments. The neuron system of the gut is a large network, second to our brain. Anyone suffering with gut pain can attest to this. The brain in our gut is an active neurotransmission, serotonin-producing system with highly intelligent messaging systems. Our digestion is intimate with every part of our physiology—as are our microbes.

## *Digestive System: Simple Basic Overview of Organs*

Digestion begins with thoughts of gratitude, visualization of divine digestion of a rainbow electric meal. Digestion begins with our connection to Mother Earth …grounded, grateful, growing, then into our mouth with quiet, plentiful mastication and thoughts of Mmmm …and thank-you, stopping at 70% full.

The Dalai Lama tells us to live like children—eat when we are hungry, sleep when we are tired and laugh all the time.

Imagine …

## *Nasal / The Mouth*

> *The mouth is the place to exercise our freedom, through breathing, talking, chanting, eating, and drinking. To manage the mouth is to manage your life properly.*

> *Michio Kushi*

Our nasal cavity is our first line of defence. Nasal is the beginning of our protective mucus membrane from the outside world. Some airborne pathogens, finding their way to your bowels thought the nasal passages, may take up residence in our small intestine creating such turbulence as small bacterial overgrowth. There's been many links between the industrial pollution we breathe and multiple diseases, including childhood asthma, multiple sclerosis, and IBD.

My old Finnish father, while visiting, commented on the oil refinery smell which all us locals get so used to smelling, "Smells like money to me!" IBD is very high per capita in this oil industrial community, once deemed industrial zone.

If we do not learn to nasal breathe as a child or we are always stuffed up from mucus forming foods such as dairy and sugar, our entire intrinsic biology suffers.

## Mouth

The food journey begins in our oral cavity, Thirty-two small bone-like structures, your teeth are called dentons. Three sets of salivary glands secrete digestive enzymes so chewing your food and your smoothies is essential for maximum digestion.

The tongue is a powerful organ for taste, gripping and pushing your food posterior for swallowing. Chewing 30–60 times takes the burden off the digestive tract since our stomach doesn't have teeth. Improper oral hygiene has been linked to heart disease and increased inflammation. A person's level of health is easily detected by the health of the teeth.

Mercury poisoning from fillings and food has been linked to heavy metal poisoning throughout the body. A healthy oral biome is of essence to oral health. The mouth also can reflect the level of body inflammation.

## The Pharynx

The pharynx and the esophagus also play a vital role in the respiratory system as air from the nasal cavity passes through the pharynx on its way to the larynx (windpipe), which goes to the lungs. The epiglottis is a flap of tissue that acts as a switch to route food to the esophagus and air to the larynx. A healthy thyroid gland, with adequate iodine, rests in this area of our throat and is the satellite centre for endocrine health.

## Esophagus

The esophagus is a muscular tube that connects the pharynx to the stomach. At the inferior end of the esophagus is a muscular ring known as the esophageal sphincter. The function of the sphincter is to close the end of the esophagus and trap food in the stomach. This is the home of acid reflux, created from acid food and acid thoughts, lack of hydrochloric acid (HCL).

## Stomach

The stomach is a muscular sac located on the left side of the abdominal cavity. The stomach is approximately the size of two fists placed next to each other and contains HCL and digestive enzymes in an acidic environment that help in the further digestive breakdown that began in the mouth. The stomach often stores excess worry.

## Liver

The liver is an accessory organ located to the right side of the stomach just lower than the diaphragm, and is approximately three pounds. The liver is an amazing organ. It performs over a hundred functions and when we do not eliminate completely even one day, our liver is forced to accumulate some of the toxins. When my bowels were tired and enervated, (meaning the nerves were tired from over-firing), I was running to the bathroom frequently but not releasing much except blood and mucus. This is important to understand, frequent urges do not equate to release of toxic waste. The liver's main function is the production of bile secretion into the small intestine; bile salts along with the gallbladder aid in the breakdown of fat. This is the main organ assisting in the detoxification process, amino acid synthesis, and decomposition of red blood cells. The liver often stores excess anger.

## Gallbladder

The gallbladder is a small pear shaped organ posterior to the liver and uses, stores and recycles excess bile from the small intestines, aids in fat digestion by releasing bile salt, and releases bile into the duodenum to break down fat. Many people with digestive issues have a weakened system and may not assimilate or breakdown fat.

## Pancreas

The pancreas is the largest gland located just inferior and posterior to the stomach; approximately six inches long, secretes enzymes leaving amino acids in their free form. It also secretes digestive enzymes into the small intestines. The pancreas malfunctions when people try to get the "sweetness" from life artificially, instead of from God, nature, love.

## Small Intestine

The small intestine is a 10-foot intestinal tract, one-inch in diameter, in the lower gastrointestinal tract that takes up most of the space in the abdominal cavity diverse in Lactobacillus. Ninety percent of all nutrients are extracted from the food in the small intestines and directed into the blood capillaries and blood stream.

Many people with IBD have small intestinal bacterial overgrowth (SIBO) and Candida. Absence of commensal bacteria has been known to cause gut dysbiosis, malabsorption, and fatigue; yet is also a main production home for glutathione, our main producers of antioxidants for detoxification. Many believe our antioxidants come from sources like blueberries; yet in fact, 85% of our glutathione is made endogenously—in our body, from our body. A healthy gut is a great contributor.

IBD is considered an autoimmune disease caused by dysregulation and hyper-immune response to the host microbiome. Microbiome researchers are challenging this definition as studies indicate people with IBD have a higher rate of firmicutes and depletion of bacteroides, (often associated with heavy animal product diets and minimal fibre), and a depletion of diversity of beneficial bacteria, along with SIBO.

People with IBD and IBS also show elevated levels of cortisol and proinflammatory cytokines IL6 and IL8. Yet simply, the intervention of probiotics such as *Lactobacillus salivarius* and *Bifidobacterium infantis* have normalized inflammation levels.[27]

## Large Intestine

The large intestine is a large thick tube approximately five feet in length. It wraps around the superior and lateral borders of the small intestine. The large intestine absorbs water and contains many symbiotic bacteria that aid in the breakdown of waste and absorption. Feces in the large intestine exit the body through the anal canal.

Absorption of simple molecules, like water and alcohol, directs immediately into the bloodstream. Although most absorption takes place in the small intestine, the large intestine is involved in the absorption of water, and vitamins B and K, before feces leave the body.

Bile salts/acid, such as glycine-conjugated cholic acid and taurine that regulate lipids, glucose, and energy, which are active in the large intestines, have been shown to be altered and degraded in their ability to function in germ-free rodents, and are influenced by diet and medication.[28]

The intestinal wall has a layer of connective tissue that holds in place the blood vessels and collects what is absorbed. Another concentric layer is the muscle cells, that through peristalsis, transport intestinal digestive chyme. When the intestines breed inflammation and are subjected to constant assault from allergens and toxins, dysfunction in the peristaltic wave and apana,(downward energy), result.[28]

In between is a discontinuous layer of immune system cells and a multitude of bacteria. Tiny nerve fibres touch the intestinal walls of the digestive tract, directing and regulating functions such as peristalsis. Contraction, timing, and strength of this action is all governed by the nerve filaments. The neuron system of the gut is a large network, second to your brain. Anyone suffering with gut pain can attest to this. The brain in our gut is an active neurotransmission, serotonin-producing system with highly intelligent messaging systems.

**What we don't eliminate, we recirculate**. This includes toxic substances we put on our skin: make-up, cleaning supplies, air fresheners… Therefore, if you cannot eat it, do not put it on your skin, or use it for cleaning, or breathe it or use it at all!! The body has to use its energy stores to detoxify it. Our skin is porous and absorbs chemicals in water and body "not so beauty" products which puts a burden on our bowels.

These are the transit times of food and liquid: water, 0–10 minutes; juice, 15–30 minutes; melon which is best not mixed with other fruit, 30–60 minutes; other fruit, 30-60 minutes; sprouts, 1 hour; most veggies,1–2 hours; grains & beans, 1-2 hours.

The bowels are the main detoxification organ along with the skin, respiratory system (breath), and urinary tract. Getting the toxins out is essential! No one can give you the experience of how good it feels to be clean. Now the misunderstanding is because one has diarrhea one is "cleaned out." An indicant bowel toxicity test will often indicate otherwise.

The primary nutrients that feed the digestive system are: vitamins A, C, B Complex, B1, B2, B6, D, E, F, K, folic acid, inositol, niacin, pantothenic acid, Mineral, sodium, chlorine, magnesium, potassium, iron, sulphur, copper, silicon, zinc, and iodine. *From Nature's Plan*, by Cheat and Jensen.

## Digestion Questions to Ponder

Am I hungry?

What would I be feeling if I wasn't eating?

Does this look and taste fresh, clean and healing?

Is this an anti-inflammatory, anti-mucus-forming food choice?

Is there something else my body needs instead of food? (Sleep, five minutes of meditation, water) Is this a "does no harm" diet choice?

Is this a conscious food choice that helps create a more aware, connected, and peaceful world? Will this food or drink bring me closer to my essence?

Am I willing to live with fragmentations of myself due to choices which contribute to suffering?

# *Bowel to Lung to Skin: Do You Read Me?*

Our skin is our most visual representation of how our system, including our bowels, are doing. But all bowel issues do not always reveal themselves through the skin. The culture of separateness treats skin disorders like acne with drugs such as minocycline and topical salicylic acid, which have many harsh side effects.

In Chinese medicine, the skin is related to the lungs and large intestine and can carry sadness. Perhaps our SAD diets and disconnect can no longer be hidden? It may be time to see detox organs such as liver, skin, bowels, lungs, and kidneys as needing to, sweat, fast, laugh, move, and hydrate, lessening the detox load. This takes some of the work off our bowels, helping significantly in reducing inflammation.

Sunlight and skin, a divine combination when not overdone, serve the vital role of vitamin D and its hormone effect. Sunlight on the skin helps assimilate D vitamins from cholesterol, lowers blood sugar by helping to metabolize it, and stimulates capillaries in bringing increased circulation to the skin. These heal skin disorders, increase mineralization, destroy *Candida*, and can strengthen our digestion by increasing our internal fire. Sunlight on the skin assists in whole-person healing.

Actor Woody Harrelson says his skin cleared when he stopped eating dairy. He then went vegan. He tells us in his documentary *Go Further*, "pus and blood" is what is in dairy. Some may find this worthy of investigating.

When our gut is inflamed and has lost integrity, it can show in the health of our skin.

# *The Cardiovascular / Respiratory / Lymphatic System*

> *For this is a great secret; all the healing forces reside originally in the human breathing system.*
>
> *~ Rudolf Steiner*

The cardiovascular system includes the heart and circulatory system. These vessels are transporters of oxygen, blood, hormones and nutrients throughout the entire body electric. A teacher of mine says that more people die of a broken heart than anything else. Without feeling the universal heart, we build plaque much more easily and we become hardened to the world, so to speak, stopping the flow.

Organs of respiration are the lungs, bronchi, trachea, larynx, pharynx and mouth. The exchange of oxygen and carbon dioxide from the chlorophyll plant world is our gift. As vegans, we are contributing significantly to save our oxygen-producing forests. Plant chlorophyll builds blood. It is often a much faster blood-builder than red meat or supplements.

We also know that plant life gives off the most oxygen during the night, especially at sunrise. We can nurture ourselves through breath during our morning walk.

The lymphatic system runs alongside our circulatory system, draining waste and destroying cells through macrophages. The lymph system moves when we move so we must rebound, massage, dry brush and keep moving to clean our lymphatics!

## So the questions we may ponder:

Why can people sun dance for days with no food and little water without collapsing?

How it is a yogi sun gazer can receive his energy from the sun for over 300 days without food?

How do we live on water for days and still walk around? Why do we often feel better after a few days on a green juice cleanse?

How do we begin to see ourselves again as WHOLE/HOLY?

Can we see how every bacteria, cell, organ and system deeply communicate in the journey of wellness?

How do we keep our hearts open and be well?

Does loving ourselves matter enough?

Why does just a 4-minute workout that releases nitric oxide make such a difference?

## STORY:

A meditation teacher, who had suffered with CD for many years, started training in yoga and meditation. He discovered, early on, that daily practice of breath and postures that developed concentration led to decreased gut symptoms. Fast-forward seven years later: he has become a healthy and mostly symptom-free practitioner of mindfulness.

## Meditation:

Listen to your body and allow yourself to move into a posture comfortable for you.

Expand the breath and movement to a comfortable edge, expanding one's patterns.

Bring consciousness to anywhere in your body, relieve tension through breath.

Keep self-aligning the posture as long as you feel expanding release.

Continue your intuitive yoga as long as your body and space-time continuum allows.

## Gratitude:

I AM grateful for the understanding of my anatomy, physiology and universal connection as ONE.

I AM an ever-changing body electric, and what I focus on, I become.

I AM electric, and drinking plenty of electron-rich water helps me cleanse and stay expansive.

I AM …

## Coming Homework:

Develop, integrate, and soar in your prana practice of belly breathing, yogic movement, Chi Nei Tsang, (unwinding the belly—worthy of study) and meditation into a conscious life.

Study which organs support bowel health and detoxification.

Smile into your organs—smiling qigong.

*If you*
*want to be able*
*to have sensitivity*
*& to feel gratitude,*
*& to have peace of mind,*
*improve your gut microbiome*

*~ Dr. Kellman*

# Chapter 9:

## *The Mysterious Microbiome & the Vagus Nerve*

### A section of science and ancient wisdom

*Counting the genes and bacteria for the 23,000 genes you have, there are 3.3 million genes that come from the microbiome*

*~ Deepak Chopra*

*The three pounds of microbes that you carry around with you might be more important than every single gene you carry around in your genome.*

**Rob Knight, biologist and co-founder**

**of the** *Human Microbiome Project.*

## 11 Microbiome Builders

1. Honour thyself and thy 100-Trillion microbial friends and fungi galore

2. De-stress (switching a stressful thought to one of gratitude instantly resets)

3. Re-inoculate in crawling around in ecosystems—swamp to sea

4. Release the war on bacteria

5. Eat to live

6. Eat plant fibre prebiotics

7 Eat from organic, veganic, living soil

8. Use herbs to support the healing of the microbiome and reduce mycotoxicity

9. Spend time on the microbial-rich earth (earthing)

10. Support natural childbirth

11. Use antibiotics as the very last option

# Gratitude & the Microbiome

Throughout this book, it is my hope that you practice keeping gratitude as an antidote to stress—cultivating thankfulness as a very fast stress reducer.

In one of the first studies of its kind and reported in *Health Psychology*, 144 people with IBD and 163 people with arthritis completed a six-month follow up survey linking the variables of gratitude with perceived stress and depression. This study revealed that gratitude remained a significant predictor of remission, lowering depression, and had a positive impact on well-being. Participants said gratitude lowered depression and sadness.[29]

# The Digestive Bacteria Tract

The 100 trillion microorganisms that hold the structural integrity of our gut and assist in metabolic functions through intestinal mucosa are paramount in keeping balanced homeostasis and maintenance of a healthy gut. Its a microbiome super warehouse: synthesizer of nutrients; a signalling network, immune regulator; and epithelial cell mediation. As the forgotten satellite organ, it is quantifying the ancient science of "all healing begins in gut health." This study is of paramount interest, and offers hopeful perspectives, yet to be fully understood, of the many roles of the microbiome in restoring endocrine function and brain health.

I suppose important questions that we need to be asking ourselves due to the state of toxicity on our planet: what are our missing microbes, and what do we do on a daily basis that manipulates and changes them within a few short hours?

Commensal bacteria has been known to stimulate epithelial cell growth and protect us from pathogenic bacteria. The microbiome signals and regulates immune system and inflammatory responses. Besides producing short-chain fatty acids (SCFAs), bacterial species of the intestinal microbiome synthesizes amino acids and vitamins (e.g., K, B12, biotin, folate, and thiamine).[30]

## Immunity: Our Microbiota

Our microbiome, our largest immune system, otherwise referred to as Gut Associated Lymphatic Tissue (GALT) is the most significant part of our immunity stimulating IgA secretion and inhibiting colonization of the GIT by pathogens. These 100 trillion bacterial cells outnumbering human cells 10:1, has been a turnaround in science's idiopathic disease model. They are epigenetic in nature. Research has indicated that microbiome health / diversity may be our way out of this health crisis epidemic and sick-care system.

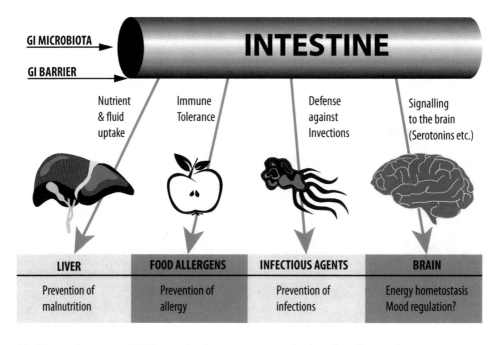

(Springernature.com, 2011) www.springernature.com/us/products/journals

As Dr. Raphael Kellman, research doctor, microbiome expert, and author of *The Microbiome Diet,* says: "Studying the microbiome is the greatest medical turnaround in 150 years." He noted that when bacteria are good and united, they create a profound "themselves" as a whole, meaning the bacteria within the host have a unified field of their own, such as the DNA cells of our body. As Yeshua was created from the dust of the earth within the microbial mystery, we are one planet, one biome.

These primordial bacteria may hold the key and have the ability to upgrade our DNA imprint. Our loss of diversity of commensal life may be what is contributing to our cultural forgetting.

Researchers out of Case Western Reserve University School of Medicine, University Hospitals Cleveland Medical Centre, and Harvard Medical School

> …tracked nitric oxide secreted by gut bacteria inside tiny worms (C. elegans, a common mammalian laboratory model). Nitric oxide secreted by gut bacteria attached to thousands of host proteins, completely changed a worm's ability to regulate its own gene expression.

> The study is the first to show gut bacteria can tap into nitric oxide networks ubiquitous in mammals, including humans. Nitric oxide attaches to human proteins in a carefully regulated manner–a process known as S-nitrosylation–and disruptions are broadly implicated in diseases such as Alzheimer's, Parkinson's, asthma, diabetes, heart disease, and cancer.[34]

# The Microbiome Role
# & Vagus Nerve Pathway

"Scientists have so far identified some ten thousand species of microbes and, because each microbe contains its own DNA, that translates to more than eight million genes. In other words, for every human gene in your body, there are at least 360 microbiome ones." ~ Dr. Perlmutter.[39]

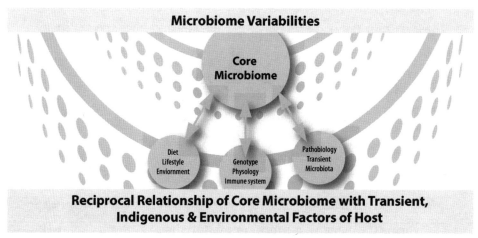

**Microbiome Variabilities**

**Core Microbiome**

Diet Lifestyle Enviornment

Genotype Physology Immune system

Pathobiology Transient Microbiota

**Reciprocal Relationship of Core Microbiome with Transient, Indigenous & Environmental Factors of Host**

The microbiome is a living matrix of mystery—dynamic and bio individual in nature. This ever changing, microscopic, non-human organism, when treated with nutrition, respect and reverence, may assist in maintaining optimal health, may ward off infection and disease, and may literally make us feel good.

It is very intriguing to imagine that 90% of our cells are non-human —90% of them are microbes and bacteria—that thrive or struggle in our gastrointestinal tract. We may be moving towards challenging the war against bacteria, to befriend and feed these bacteria that will accompany us in doing everything from digesting food, regulating appetite, controlling metabolism, and balancing our immunity, to creating elevated moods (for up to 90% of serotonin, our feel good hormone is produced in the intestines with the assistance of microbes).

Dr. Alessio Fasano of Harvard calls these gut bacteria signals from the immune cells our body's "first responders." In this responding mechanism, the gut will either release inflammation or stress molecules or in a healthy gut, do the opposite.[31]

There are only four nucleotides in DNA that respond to the majority of life on this planet. The bacteria are the masters of those four nucleotides. They control the software of our microbiome, a complete interconnected system, no separation. Perhaps, through our microbiota we will be able to deepen our connection to the Oneness.

The commonly accepted germ theory and war on bacteria through antibiotics and vaccines has minimum application toward our understanding that diversity and balance of our gut bacteria provides resiliency to potentially harmful viruses/bacteria. It is now widely known that healthy gut bacteria = health. Looking through this new lens, we see even viruses in a new light! That the measles virus protects us against diseases, such as atopy in children. In the words of GreenMedInfo founder Sayer Ji: "These viruses are a piece of the genetic code, searching for a chromosome."

## Brain Health & Stress Release is in the Gut

Gastroenterologist, researcher, and author of *The Gut Mind Connection*, Emeran Mayer, states: "It becomes clear that gut microbes have an extensive and wholly unexpected influence on the appetite-control and emotional operating systems in your brain, on your behaviour and even your minds; your gut-based decisions and how your brain develops and ages."[32]

Our processed and cultural "forgetting" about real food and vital microbes has some of us searching for our missing microbes of peace and sanity.

Some of the original work by Lyte and Ernst in 1992–1997, in the field of microbial endocrinology, explains how stress-induced neuroendocrine hormones have a direct influence on pathogenic bacterial growth while signalling neurotoxins. This research has increased our knowledge about how stressors may alter microbe composition rapidly.[33]

Most diseases appear to have their origin in the gut. This understanding appears to be the root exploratory pathway in the BIG question: considering how IBD, diabetes, arthritis, cancer, obesity and brain disorders are on the rise and, viewed through the lens of microbiome research, appear to have a systemic link to our individual diet, exposure to herbicides, pesticides, antibiotics and pathogens as well as stress, surgery, microbiota early development, and lost connection to this microbial rich earth: would it not be wise to look here first?

Our living ecology is suffering, more contaminants than ever are seen on the planet—many through the byproducts of animal agriculture and food grown for animal consumption.

*In the words of Dr. Larry Dossey in* One Mind, *If I had to pinpoint the most valuable lesson that may come out of the microbiome, I think it's the lesson that we cannot separate from nature and, by us trying to do that, it has left us in a precarious position on this planet.*

We are no longer able to overlook this connection. So how do we befriend our hundred trillion friendly bacteria? These non-human microbes are amazingly simple and complex at the same time. Some can thrive in freezing temperatures and others in boiling temperatures. Some can tolerate radiation and they feast on everything imaginable, from sugar and fibre to sunlight and air. Absolutely nothing can exist without them and when the diversity and beneficial microbes die, so do we. Perhaps reviewing our reconnection to original and beneficial microbes, and our responsibility to co-evolve on this planet may be the shortcut home.

The microbiome is a language with incredible organization, with 16,000 bacteria alone required just to break down carbohydrate.[34]

Bacteria and microbes are necessary for every enzymatic process and nourishment absorption that the body requires. The microbiome is even a producer of natural antibiotics. Within this inner garden, we will either set up sugar-craving cycles or feed this ecology pre and probiotic-rich foods such as plant fibre, sauerkraut, seed, organic/veganic, and low pathogenic bacteria plant food. These cultured foods may possibly completely alter and release our disease/food addictions.

The bacteria *bifidobacterium*, for example, have the ability to generate vitamins such as K, B12, biotin, thiamine and folate. *Lactobacillus, Bacteroides*, and *Bifidobacterium* mediate lipid transports in the turnover of human cells.[35]

Through balancing, healing and honouring our microbiome, people have reversed illnesses: severe candida, autoimmune disorders, autism and various metabolic symptoms such as obesity and diabetes as demonstrated in the work of Donna Gates in *The Ecology Diet*, Dr. Campbell McBride in *Gut and Psychology Syndrome* and Donna Schwenk in *Cultured Food for Life*.[20,36,37]

Bonnie Bassler, microbiologist, shares how our 100 trillion single cell bacteria talk to each other. In her TED Talk, *How Bacteria Talk*, she gives the example of *Vibrio Fischeri*—which are the bioluminescent bacteria that we see in the oceans. In low density, they do not produce light, but when a quorum of minimal numbers are formed, luminescence is made under the light of the moon. This is called dilute suspension. They literally talk to each other asking, "are there enough of us yet?" and if not, they lay dormant, splitting down the centre and reproducing until enough have been made and, through chemical communication, they are able to complete their job. In this quorum sensing, bacteria can distinguish between self and others. They know both pathogenic and bacteria of the self; hence, pathogenic bacteria lay dormant if the self-bacteria is too great a number for the pathogenic quorum to invade. This is how we, the bacteria, make harmful bacteria benign.[38]

*I'm a WANDERER: VAGUS*

*Wandering, vagus wanderer*
*What do you seek?*
*Your happy, healing, calming microbes?*

*Are you stressing out with the germ theory, endless hurry, antibiotics,*
*glyphosate and C-sections galore …*
*Leaving, searching the cosmos for more,*
*something missing from deep within.*
*Oh sweet wanderer, what are you longing for?*

*The war on microbes*
*The war raging within*
*The war against others*
*Where did it begin?*

*The fire in the belly*
*Inflamed angry wander "Oh, the nerve!"*
*Is it going to your head?*
*The war on microbes*
*Imbedded deep induced fear*

*YET…*

*Gardens of Peace*
*The cosmos in a carrot*
*The universe in a dish*
*Peace gardens coming home*
*Alive soil to table Rebirth*
*Inoculated with happy microbes …*

*Oh wandering one, what are you searching for?*
*Is it your microbes …*
*In the puppies, grass, water*
*Structured and pure?*
*Is it 'Effective Microorganisms' to heal all other "isms"?*
*Is it in ION\*Bione galore?*

*HERE IT IS!*
*In the missing microbes' spore*
*In the yogi's silent listening*
*Ancient deities calling us home…*

*And from the heart of Rumi, we will remember "what we are seeking,*
*is seeking us"*

# *Oh You Vagus—The Nerve!*

Vagus from the Latin root "vaga" meaning to wander, is the longest of the twelve cranial nerves, known as the 10th cranial nerve, rooted deep in our abdomen and extending all the way up to our brainstem, wandering over to our lungs and heart, seeking all organ-ic connection. It works on the ANS, meaning our nervous systems are directly affected by the bacteria in our guts. The stimulation that is created from our gut microbes controls chemical messengers along this wandering nerve pathway. It extends into our brain with its own enteric nervous system, generating many of the same neurotransmitters—serotonin and acetylcholine interactions, and reacting to every organ system.[39]

This bidirectional communication system, which includes both our ENS and ANS, is richly nourished with vascular beds, Peyer's patches, and T lymphocytes.

There is a 9:1 ratio of afferent nerves, compared to efferent nerve bundles, that supply our intestines. Our guts are controlling our brains. What we feed it matters, be it love food, fear or other anxiety-laden food! This vagal nerve supply equates to 30,000 to 80,000 nerve bundles carrying information to our brain, compared to a small fraction of nerves that return information to our gut. It is our intestines that are directing our brain in what to do, not the otherway around.[40]

This second brain, through the vagus stimuli, has the ability to control hormones, regulate muscle movement and act as the warehouse to the largest part of our immune system.[28]

Research tells us that we tone-stimulate this nerve through and through by:

1. Yoga
2. Singing, chanting, toning

3. Cold water and cold face washing
4. Deep relaxation
5. Stretching
6. Deep, baby belly breathing
7. Nutrition
8. Massage
9. Gratitude, as it reduces stress instantly

In an abstract titled "Vagal, On Pathways For Microbiome-Brain-Gut Access Communication," it was found:

> There's strong evidence from studies that gut microorganisms can activate the vagus nerve, and that such activation plays a critical role in mediating effects on the brain and behaviour. The vagus appears to differentiate between non-pathogenic and potentially pathogenic bacteria, even in the absence of overt inflammation. [41]

The microbiome-brain-gut axis communication, via the vagus nerve, has the ability to:

- Turn on anti-inflammatory responses

- Release mediators, such as acetylcholine, that interact with immune cells

- Play an immune modulating role initiating from the vagus nerve, which has been shown to also modulate mood and brain function. It appears research is moving toward looking at nutritional stimuli and the gut-brain implications to heal both depression and mood disorders.[41]

*Most of the metabolites are not coming*
*from our cells; they are coming from our gut microbes*

*~ Dr. Kellman*

Most people with gut inflammation feel sad and irritable. Professor Bernstein in the department of Gastroenterology at the University of Manitoba discovered that mood disorders always precede gut problems. He went on to explain that having bacteria in your bowel triggers an immune response that also impacts brain function. "By manipulating the bugs in the bowel, one may be able to improve mood disorders."

The brain has over 100 billion neurons, whereas the gut has close to 500 million nerve cells that send electrical signals via the vagus nerve and chemical reactions through the blood-brain. The neural network is used in various ways through the complex reaction of digestion, absorption, muscle contraction and all the other autonomic gut reactions that work interconnected with the brain.[19]

Our personal biochemistry may be beneficially altered through healthy influences of our gut's microbiome; our dopamine/serotonin manufacturer. The gut's microbiota brain appears to be involved directly with development, behaviour and mood. The microbiota is now well recognized for its interplay with diet, stress, and the treatment of mental health and metabolic disorders.

Dr. Perlmutter, in *Brain Maker*, states: "Scientific research is bringing more and more credence to the notion that up to 90% of all non-human illness can be traced back to an unhealthy gut."[19]

In 2014 the U.S. National Institute for Mental Health spent one million dollars on new research to study the gut microbiome and the brain. They discovered the vagus nerve was the connector to the brain in digestive immunity—enriched with beneficial bacteria. Now mental illnesses are being viewed through a microbial lens: i.e. healthy fecal microbiota transplants in anxious mice have a dramatic calming effect after only one transplant, as do probiotics and dietary changes.

The link between stress and inflammatory flare-ups is irrefutable. No matter what is going on, we have the ability to bring ourselves into a calmer state through breath-work and gratitude. Dr. Vincent Pedre, in *Happy Gut*, also shares this understanding, that gratitude is always the antidote for stress. He has found in his research as a functional doctor that he has had the greatest success in patients who understand this. The two cannot symbiotically take up residence in the mind. As true as this may be, the question remains: does a diet that builds commensal bacteria symbiotically increase calmness and allow easier access to gratitude?

The microbe expression has also been seen to enhance tryptophan production which is a precursor for serotonin, improving sleep, mood, and anxiety levels. In studies by researcher Desbonnet, *Bifidobacterium infantis* has been known to combat psychosis with its neurotransmitter effect. It is one of the first probiotics of the infant and may be lacking when a child is not breastfed. As mentioned earlier, 90% of serotonin is located in the GI tract of the enterochromaffin cell. The responsibility of these cells, in the release of serotonin, is to stimulate LPS and enzymes, that help in the detoxification of toxins.[27]

It appears new levels of peace, connection and liberation may be reached when gut-brain-metabolic bacteria are diverse, we are nutritionally sound, have vitamin/minerals available, and the bowels are cleared of toxic waste. It is liberating and hopeful that we can change gut composition of transient bacteria quite quickly.

Yet just glyphosate alone destroys our bacteria shikimate pathway and alkaloid medicines in food, which are anticancer and antiasthmatic. Conventional chemical farming also disrupts essential amino acids of tryptophan and tyrosine, which are the building blocks that promote our ability to sleep and build.

*"The connection between Earth's vast ecosystems of bacteria, fungi, parasites, and viruses, and human health is extraordinary. The pharmaceutical model of human health and disease has convinced so many of us that the microbial world is our enemy. From flu to Lyme ...from parasites to small bowel bacterial overgrowth ...we believe our species to be at odds with the microbiome. Yet, our efforts to fight or manipulate the microbiome (vaccines, antibiotics, and probiotics) undermine our health."*

*Dr. Zach Bush, M.D.*

We do know a healthy gut microbiome is needed in this synthesis of nutrition.

In research studying the importance of fermentation within the large bowel and healthy GI tract, carbohydrates and dietary fibre of not less than 27 grams per day showed to be therapeutic in the treatment of IBD cardiovascular disease and Type 2 diabetes. Organic acids, as the byproduct of fermentation, provide energy for the bowels' peripheral tissues and epithelium cells—as SCFA being the major end product. SCFA stimulated sodium-coupled transportation of water and electrolyte synthesis.[4]

There is this fast/slow paradox: the stress of a fast-paced world, fast food, a hyper mind and an overstimulated soul leads to a slow brain and body, and rapid deterioration of beneficial bacteria. I have mostly eaten well in my life. I have loved vegetables and fruit from my beginning of time. I was told that the seeds of Crohn's began 10 days after birth when my mother was taken to the hospital with a blood clot that was heading to her brain. I went from nursing on breast-milk to drinking diluted carnation evaporated milk. As the story goes, I cried endlessly.

Throughout my life well into adulthood, I would fluctuate from mostly being constipated to diarrhea, despite my high-fibre diet. When my stress came to an all-time high in my early 40s, I began to develop first mucus, then blood, in my stool. Within only three weeks of following live-food organic diet, juicing and various treatments at the *Hippocrates Health Institute*, (such as wheatgrass, chlorophyll-rich juicing, and pureed salads, hydrotherapy, mindbody love focus), then healing happened fast. The terrain was favourable!

With these higher amounts of animal fats, we see an increased amount of what is often known as the fat-inducing microbe: firmicutes and proteobacteria.

Find peace within food as medicine. Befriend food once again. **Joy began, as it turned out, more in my gut than in my head.**

## *STORY:*

My son died a young man, in 2017, of a heart condition. I was able to witness firsthand how quickly he started feeling better after arriving home, often directly from ICU, when his diet consisted of green juice and whole plant-based food, mostly raw. Yet coping strategies and broken hearts die hard.

Our bodies are incredible self-healing organisms. There is much speculation on whether my son had an undiagnosed genetic issue, or how much lifestyle came into play, or whether, due to some of his early experiences, his inability to deal with the deep heartbreak contributed to his "broken heart syndrome."

Unravelling the history of illness is always multifaceted, yet miraculous, and often worthy of the ride. As long as humans have inhabited the earth, we have been feeling beings, sayings such as "have a heart." or "I just have a gut feeling." These have been expressions or metaphors we have used that have indicated our "three-mind" connection.

Over the last few years, research has discovered the scientific connection of all three. It appears that the heart and gut have a mind of their own—cross-talking and hearing the microbes that gather strength in numbers, speaking the loudest.

## Meditation:

Sit quietly and breathe. Feel the settling of your visceral nerves and deep abdominal nerves through breath. Understand this wandering nerve as a key messenger telling you which food, activity or practice assists your healing, or begins a cascade of stress signalling. Be grateful for this beautiful feedback system. Honour it through your actions.

## Gratitude:

I AM wandering through the diverse biomes around me in nature, contemplating my connection with health and honouring my body as the messenger.

I AM one with all breathing systems, revitalizing myself with universal microbes—each breath releasing all that no longer serves me.

I AM …

## Coming Homework

Develop the H.E.A.L protocol for your beautiful anatomy daily:

H-hydrate with 10 glasses of water, structured water from hydrating living food and raw veggie juices and herb tea daily. Heal the integrity of the gut through supplementation and living soil.

H - Homeostasis through rest, movement, connection, and nutrition

E - Energize and move every day, eat electron-rich food as spoken throughout this book.

A - Keep the body Alkaline and live an anti-inflammatory diet.

L - Move towards Love and Light, for that is all you are.

*The most beneficial way
to heal the microbiome is to
take the foot off the gas pedal and
stop feeding yeast, fungi and pathogenic food
and most importantly to
stop eating sugar
in all forms. For most people
have significant bacteria overgrowth.*

*~ Dr. Mercola*

# Chapter 10:

# *Specific Diets in Balancing the Microbiome:*

## Bacteria and Fungi—Friend or Foe Connection

*The key to restoring health is minimizing or eliminating the toxic conditions so that the composting button is turned off. A low-sweet, live food, non-acidic diet and a healthy mind are the keys to turning off the compost button and reestablishing health.*

**Dr. Gabriel Cousens**

*We have known for a long time people can get infected with viruses and bacteria and not get sick. Now we have the scientific evidence that not every viral infection is bad, but may actually be beneficial to health, just as we know that many bacterial infections are good for maintaining health.*

**Ken Cadwell, NYU University**

# Diet & the Microbiome

## 1st Diet Protocol - Organic/Authentically Grown

Our gut bacteria is the filtering lenses of every habit, choice and behaviour: both conscious and unconscious. This is moving from dis-ease to a diversity model of wellness. The ancient art of culturing foods offers us both an incredible array of prebiotics and probiotics, while increasing the bioavailability and the vitamin/mineral richness of our food. My dear friend Alex is participating in a conscious community called *New Earth* in California, where they are developing ground-regenerative cultured food. These include *Bifidobacterium* and *Lactobacillus*, which produce "a happy signal" called GABA that acts on the nervous system to curb anxiety and depression. This is the opposite effect of the negative bacteria family called Clostridium, which dines on animal fat and sugar. Part of the challenge is sticking to healthy eating long enough to clear the mental fog.[42]

Studies support this, in particular—*Effects of Regulating Intestinal Microbiota on Anxiety Symptoms in General Psychiatry*, in which twenty-one studies used a total of 1503 subjects had an 86% success rate in decreasing anxiety by changing the microbiota through diet as compared to a probiotic intervention. This research in gut-brain access has also revealed changing diet to support healthy microbiome to reduce anxiety diversity is more effective than many interventions including probiotics as supplements..[43]

# What are Mycotoxins?

## 11 Foods High in Mycotoxicity

1. SUGARS - both cane and sugar beets and even all natural sugar feeds yeast

2. COTTONSEED

3. PEANUTS

4. ALCOHOLIC BEVERAGES and COFFEE

5. WHEAT and most grains, pasta, breads, GLUTEN

6. SORGHUM

7. CHEESE

8. CORN and all corn products

9. BARLEY

10. RYE

11. ALL PROCESSED FOOD [44]

A friend sent me "breaking news" in 2017 on a CD study linking CD to Candida Tropicalis and two closely-linked bacteria. This "news flash," unknown to many, was actually first discovered by Dr. Antoine Bechamp in the 19th century as a sign we were decomposing.[11]

Dr. Robert Young explains: "We Do Not Get Old, WE MOULD"! This is seen in so many with systemic yeast and fungi infections. In Dr. Bechamp's work, he saw blood as flowing liquid tissue and discovered "microzymes," or ferments in the blood, were living microscopic elements capable of fermenting sugars in our system. Bechamp advocated for a healthier inner terrain free of mycotoxicity as a key to health. This balanced inner ecology was acutely disrupted by an acidic diet filled with sugar and acidic food and all its byproducts. Bechamp named this degeneration of our microbiome and the beginning of dysbiosis as pleomorphism.[45]

This work was further studied by Dr. Günther Enderlein and one of his students, Dr. Maria Blecker, who both concluded through blood research that protist microorganisms change form according to their environment.[45]

We all remember the line from a Beatles song, "I get by with a little help from my friends." This is also true when it comes to microbes. We would be best to heed the advice of a low mycotoxin diet, that is well researched yet not well understood, and make friends with the bacteria that love us back.

Many lifestyle factors can contribute to inflammation in our intestines. Not surprisingly, research suggests bacteria and fungi are involved in maintaining this balance. While we rely on antibiotics as a key player in preventing disease, our learning curve has been quite slow in understanding the side effects of antibiotic resistance, and the destruction that antibiotics have on microbiome health diversity. We have discovered that with issues like C.diff, Crohn's, colitis and fistulating disease, continually treating them with wide-spectrum antibiotics has prevented our microbiome from doing its job.

Much is misunderstood of the role of macronutrients when we look at health and the microbiome. Everything we eat will digest poorly when we have leaky gut. Fibre will inflame, and acidic animal products high on the toxic food chain can sink us. Let us look at a little biology: the food must be eaten by the bacteria and fungus; packaged by your "others" into the liver into blood vessels; and once taken up by the cell mitochondria, then fat and carbohydrates are turned into acetyl coA. When acetyl coA reacts with water and electron energy, then ATP is available for energy.

*If you kill the microbiome, you start into the starvation state, liver stores sugars and fats instead of sending the fuel on to the mitochondria. Obesity and insulin resistance=starvation stress at the mitochondrial level!*

**Zach Bush, MD.**

It is now, more than ever, of great importance to understand the impact of environmental toxins in the soil, air, water, and food supply, and how crucial it is to keep our internal environment detoxified from highly contaminated food and drink.

The references made by early pioneers, who studied the *Lactobacilli* strains of lactic acid in the fermentation of milk, were using what was available at the time. Nowadays, we have a consortium of plant-based options to draw upon that promote peace, love, and beneficial microbes for all.

Microbiome alterations are evident in IBS, autism and diabetes. And all patients tested who suffer with mental disorders are deficient in good flora. Many of these people often crave the gluteo-morphine effect of gluten and casein-morphine effect of dairy.[36,37]

Diets rich in plant fibre are an important part in the microbial production of short-chain, fatty acids. Many studies done on the SADs reveal that low-dietary fibre significantly decreased beneficial bacteria, which is now being recognized to be the leading cause of food cravings and addiction.

# Specific Diets Focusing on the Healing Gut

## 1. FODMAP Diet

FODMAPs are short-chain carbohydrates, sugars and alcohols found in foods naturally or as additives. FODMAPs include fructose, glucose, fructans, galacto-oligosaccharides (GOS), lactose and polyols.

A diet low in FODMAPs is scientifically proven as an effective dietary therapy for IBS and symptoms of an irritable digestion.

FODMAP is an acronym that stands for:

**Fermentable**—meaning they are broken down (fermented) by bacteria in the large bowel

**Oligosaccharides**—"oligo" means few and "saccharide" means sugar. These molecules made up of individual sugars joined together in a chain.

**Disaccharides**—"di" means two. This is a double-sugar molecule.

**Monosaccharides**—"mono" means single. This is a single-sugar molecule.

**Polyols**—these are sugar alcohols

How do FODMAPs trigger symptoms of IBS? When consumed in food and drink, they will often have a negative effect on people who have (SIBO) and will impact when the small intestine is healed from pathogenic bacteria.[46]

The FODMAPs look at fermented bacteria in the large bowel, contributing to the production of gas. I have witnessed the increase of bloating and gas when people begin to add cultured food, such as sauerkraut to their diet.

This is why it is always advised to start very slow during the time of "die-off" in the small and large intestine. For example, even one tablespoon of sauerkraut juice each day could be enough.

FODMAPs are also highly osmotic, meaning that they attract water into the large bowel, although many juice-fasters have been able to tolerate in diluted juice form. It is often the fibre in these foods that trigger the effect.

The Low FODMAP Diet is proven to be an effective dietary treatment for the vast majority of people suffering from IBS and IBD. Most of these foods are offenders on all of the diets listed below. It is wise to look at this interconnection between what each specific diet is omitting, such as all disaccharides, sugars, grain, and processed food.[46]

## 2. Specific Carbohydrate Diet

SCD, founded by Biochemist Elaine Gottschall, focuses on a monosaccharide diet that omits all grains and sugars that are disaccharides and relies on fruit, vegetables, and animal products in their unprocessed form for healing. Gottschall's diet, the Carbohydrate Specific Diet, was her PhD. work in her "mother bear" attempt to heal her dying child of colitis.

This was the first diet that I implemented for healing IBD, but with minimal results. This is understood upon researching the extremely high pathogenic bacteria count in conventional eggs, milk, and meat. The pathogens in animal products have often been the culprit of salmonella, *E.coli*, poisoning—deadly for the compromised microbiota. Milk has been known to be addictive with its casein-morphine affect; gluten with its gluteo-morphine effect.

Toxicity and the high-absorption rates of pathogenic bacteria in a person with bowel hyper-permeability explain the high recovery rate of people adopting a plant-based diet. Gottschall was seeking a cure for her young child dying from ulcerative colitis. It was when I went plant-based that I was able to experience the profound healing in my recovery with IBD. When a person is suffering with IBD, they have inflammation of the mucosa lining villi, (the finger-like projections that cover the digestive tract and help break down complex carbohydrates into simple form)which are usually flattened and damaged.[18]

## 3. The Gut and Psychology Syndrome (a.k.a. the GAPS diet)

As many people have become seekers of alternative ways to eat as a result of illness and a complete disruption of intestinal homeostasis, so it is true for GAPS founder, Dr. Natasha Campbell-McBride, who was seeking answers to her child's autism. Hence, we link the gut-brain connection once again to diet and lifestyle. Campbell-McBride and the GAPS diet takes the SCD further down the path. It understands flesh food and dairy as difficult to digest and focuses on bone broth and bowel rest to heal inflammation. Both diets are steeped in probiotic inoculation, and omitting sugar and grains for gut and brain health.[36]

## 4. The Maker's Diet

This diet, by Jordan Rubin who cured IBD in the early part of his adult life, relies on unprocessed and organic food, specific supplementation, and probiotics. He later developed The Garden of Life raw supplement line.[47]

## 5. Essene and Natural Hygiene Healing Diet

The research in this body of work, and my own body-mind-spirit, personal trials and tribulations, has shown me this is the only diet that allows me to remain in remission. This includes bowel rest, juicing, intermittent fasting, conscious eating, and mindful growing and mastication.[48, 49 50, 51]

It would be wise to note all the above diets omit sugars and grain in the acute inflammatory stage for they feed disease, and eliminate disaccharide foods that help form polysaccharides and are toxic and inflammatory to the body.

Today, much research is directed at what "normal" gut microbial communities look like and how bacteria play a role in health and disease. Throughout this and other research, it profiles that greater abundance of commensal bacteria are found in children, as well as cultures eating mostly plant-based diets such as 7th Day Adventists, who have been consuming vegan diets over a long time and have some of the healthiest communities of centenarians ever studied. We may begin to see the connection in *The Blue Zone.*[52]

Our microbiome is a neurochemical manufacturer of dopamine and serotonin. It has the ability to create disease resistance. Through healthy body, mind, and spirit, we can maintain a healthy gut lining and begin repairing metabolic syndromes.[19]

Research out of Harvard suggests gut microbes alter within two days from extreme meat and cheese diets:

> Microbial activity mirrored differences between herbivorous and carnivorous mammals, reflecting trade-offs between carbohydrate and protein fermentation. Foodborne microbes from both diets transiently colonized the gut, including bacteria, fungi and even viruses. Finally, increases in the abundance and activity of *Bilophila wadsworthia* on the animal-based diet support a link between dietary fat, bile acids and the outgrowth of microorganisms capable of triggering inflammatory bowel disease. In concert, these results

demonstrate that the gut microbiome can rapidly respond to altered diet, potentially facilitating the diversity of human dietary lifestyle.[53]

# Pathogens in Food

Animal products, including dairy, have been linked to suffering and the destruction of our ecosystem, and have been contributing factors in the spread of infectious pathogenic bacteria and viruses amongst us. Dr. Michael Greger says in Nutritionfacts.org:

> Arachidonic acid (AA)-derived eicosanoids belong to a complex family of lipid mediators that regulate a wide variety of physiological responses and pathological processes. AA have been studied and understood as creating pathological processes in autoimmunity. AA are found in all animal flesh.[53]

In the following article on the Advantages of the health benefits of a vegan diet, Glick-Bauer, Ming-Shin, and Yeh note:

> The vegan gut profile appears to be unique in several characteristics, including a reduced abundance or pathobionts and a greater abundance of protected species. Reduced levels of inflammation, may be the key feature linking the vegan gut microbiota with protective health effects… the twenty-one vegans were found to have lower blood pressure and lower fasting triacylglycerols and glucose concentrations than twenty-five omnivore subjects, as well as biochemical profiles that were cardio-protective and beta cell-protective.[54]

This research also concluded that inflammasomes, which are a group of protein complexes that create inflammation-inducing stimuli and are responsible for metabolic diseases, have been regulated and altered into symbiotic commensal bacteria through a plant-based diet. The vegan gut profile has a reduced amount of the pathogenic bacteria *Enterobacteriaceae* and shows a more abundant protective species of *F.prausnitzii*. The research helps clarify the limited concept of veganism.[54]

Pleomorphism, according to Webster's dictionary, means "many forms of the body." It is the ability of bacteria to change into colonies that are commensal or pathogenic. It appears that much of this is done through how we control the blood pH. The microorganism can transform so much that it can resemble a virus more than a bacteria.

Dr. Robert Young states:

> Involved in the concept of pleomorphism was the role and importance of the host organism—THE PATIENT! Microbes altered their forms in response to the patient, in response to the diet, environmental stresses the patient encountered, what poisons the patient consumed etc." …The patient had control over the bacteria, not the other way around. The micro-form found in the body is the result, not the cause of dis-ease or so-called disease. Even the common so-called "communicable" diseases, e.g. strep throat or chickenpox, cannot take hold, grow if the internal milieu is not conducive to their reproduction or growth.[45]

John Phillips, who taught Conscious Veganic Gardening at the *Tree of Life Rejuvenation Centre*, invites us to see pleomorphism on a grander cosmic scale. He tells us that we share more DNA with a mushroom than any other plant. Through his work with "effective microorganisms," we begin to understand bacteria as a healthy way to coexist rather than bacteria as an antagonist.[16]

The understanding of pleomorphism puts the responsibility back on each of us, as well as farmers and the communities, as we grow food to clean up our water and resources, regaining sovereignty and wisdom.

**The questions that remain are:**

- What microbes are we feeding?

- What is eating us?

- How will that make us who we are? Such as, when we feed our microbes sugar, *Candida albicans*, which lives in most of us, can pleomorphism into a full-blown yeast infection that can inhabit and weaken our whole body.

- What are your microbes telling you and how does your everyday diet affect your gut reaction and intuition?

- Who is eating whom?

- Is what we're feeding our bacteria beneficial or not?

- Can we eventually overcome peer pressure, both internally and externally through what we feed ourselves?

- If most of our bacteria (90-99%) are good bacteria in a healthy host, then is it best to get the LIVING probiotics in place, allowing it to be incredibly simple to avoid the few invaders?

- How do we support the "die-off" cravings of yeast, lessening the impact?

In the early stages of disease, many people display an increased number of pathogenic microbes of yeast, parasites, and fungi. The compromised mucosa barrier creates hyper permeability, allowing undigested food particles to pass into the bloodstream, which often triggers increased allergen responses. Ingestion of anything, no matter how minuscule, can exacerbate inflammation and the detox response. It becomes very evident at this time that what we do not ingest may be of equal or greater value to what nutrition we are adding.

Ulceration, inflammation, and all the side effects of an inflamed gut—flatulence and abdominal distention, fluctuating with diarrhea and constipation and the release of mucous—are all acute stages of an inner ecology out of balance.

Beneficial bacteria have been shown to allow the protective biofilm of the intestines to support healing. In a compromised epithelial mucosa lining, continuing to create insult (allergens) will continue permeating the mucosa immunity barrier.

Most common allergens are dairy, sugar, and animal products, and all disaccharide chemically farmed foods; such as grain, corn, gluten and simple sugars that have double sugars and require a healthy mucosa lining to break down. The secret is there is no secret. Our gut flora flourishes in the absence of sugar, moulds, yeasts and acid, and thrives in a clean-living alkaline, and highly mineralized electron diet.

Former World Health Organization researcher, Dr. A.V. Costantini, found that people with Crohn's often have aflatoxin, a mycotoxin made by *Aspergillus* moulds, in their blood. And, according to Dr. Mercola, research seems to confirm the potential role of aflatoxin in Crohn's, as disease activity in patients with Crohn's was lower while they followed a yeast-free diet, specifically avoiding baker's and brewer's yeasts. In the same research, it was found that Crohn's patients have higher amounts of the bacteria *Serratia marcescens* and *E. coli* in their intestines, along with the fungus Candida tropicalis. Experiments revealed that these three microorganisms interact to create an inflammatory biofilm that, in turn, produces the symptoms of Crohn's.[55]

# Diet: Beyond Meat

We are in mass denial of the obvious link between meat-eating and microbial/diversity destruction, says Jeremy Rifkin in *Beyond Beef*. He gives some startling facts: livestock contributes to: more than 18% of global weather fluctuations (more than 760 million vehicles);, 60% of nitric oxide, and 30% of methane. One-third of our agriculture is harvested to feed animals and up to 70% is used to grow feed for animals. One pound of beef takes 12 pounds of feed to produce and one hamburger needs 660 gallons of water to produce.

Rifkin notes that humans, while only accounting for .05% of the biomass on earth, consume 24% of all the photosynthesis.[56]

Dr. Cousens, in *Conscious Eating*, says:

"The inhumane way in which we treat animals and "hygienically filthy" manner inspecting nine or more birds per minute and over three hundred cows per hour' leave us susceptible to E. coli poisoning that are radiation-resistant." [50]

"Contamination by foodborne pathogens and mycotoxins was examined in 475 eggs and 20 feed samples collected from three egg layer farms, three egg-processing units, and five retail markets."[57]

# Got Milk:

Milk is addictive, mucus forming and, as research shows, over 75% of people are allergic to it. Translation: it creates inflammation and toxicity. Many lifestyle factors can contribute to inflammation in our intestines. Dairy also has a scientific-proven additive substance called casein, which is known to create addictive cravings for it. Surprisingly, research suggests bacteria and fungi are involved.

Previous research has linked Crohn's disease to the presence of a bacterium called *Mycobacterium paratuberculosis*, which prevents white blood cells from killing E. coli bacteria known to be present in increased numbers within Crohn's disease-infected tissue. One route of exposure to these mycobacteria is cow's milk. Many studies link milk to inflammation and is mucus-forming, which is why singers do not consume dairy before performing. *Mycobacterium avium paratuberculosis* (MAP) was present in about 92 percent of patients with Crohn's disease, compared to 26 percent of patients in a control group. MAP is present in various percentages of commercial pasteurized milk.

Dr. Martin Blaser, in his book *Missing Microbes*, gives some startling studying on dairy poisoning. He discovered that people taking antibiotics within a month prior to drinking contaminated milk were five and a half times more likely to become ill. Healthcare professionals warned the residents that taking antibiotics would leave them more susceptible to infections, specifically salmonella. In light of the high pathogenic bacteria in animal products, would it not be wise to omit them while healing and beyond? [58]

Most dairy farms, even organic, take the new calf away from its mother immediately to direct dairy to us. Is there a direct correlation to the disconnect of family?

The concern with eating a diet high in pathogenic bacteria is the toxic load this forces the body to expel. Therefore, it is in this author's opinion that loving deeper, with education and experiences, and consuming a live-food plant-based organic diet while eliminating pathogenic food, is of paramount importance. A healthy gut can normalize some amount of pathogen, a sick leaky gut cannot.

# Gluten & Sugar

It would be wise for us to continue to look at the link between gut inflammation and systemic inflammation, such as how most people with IBD become arthritic, depressed, and systemically inflamed. When the villi on the small intestines are compromised, grains usually putrefy in the gut.

The properties of gluten are known as gluteo-morphine or gliadorphin. This is an opioid peptide, which is formed from undigested gliadin and gluten, and is highly addictive. In the case of intestinal dysbiosis, the permeability of the intestines allows those undigested molecules to enter the bloodstream and pass through the blood/brain barrier. Autistic kids and most of society appear addicted to gluten and sugar. Perlmutter, in *Grain Brain*, states: "A person may be sensitive to either of these proteins or to one of the twelve different smaller units that make up gliadin. Any could cause a sensitivity reaction leading to inflammation."[39]

This speaks of the profound influence and dependence of the brain on the gut's microbiome—as the microbiome regulates neurotransmitters and many enzymatic actions. To re-inoculate with fermented foods, grow and eat colourful high-fibre, above-ground vegetables while avoiding grains and sugar would be a wise rebuilding protocol.

Perlmutter tells the revealing truth of gluten's impact on brain inflammation and degenerative brain disease. Taoist culture has known for centuries that grain makes them foggy. Gluten is also a molecule mimicker, producing intestinal hyper-permeability, zonulin, and thyroid molecular mimicry that degrades thyroid function. People I have counselled who consume dairy or gluten also experience inflamed bowels. And if I continue treating them, my skin suffers, including cold sores.

Donna Gates, author of the *Body Ecology Diet*, is one of the pioneers in discovering core nutrients to support the gut and key principles to assist our inner ecology in healing her systemic yeast infections. Her protocol now supports healing beginnings and raising children sugar-free.[20]

Dr. Robynne Chutkan, an integrative gastroenterologist, published a study in which she took nine people with Crohn's and three people with ulcerative colitis, and removed gluten and processed sugar from their diet. The ones that added more fibre in the form of vegetables, such as green smoothies and inulin from Jerusalem artichoke, did significantly better.[28]

It has been found helpful to: re-inoculate with fermented foods, to eat colourful high-fibre, above-ground vegetables, to avoid all grain; and, starting as low as 1 TBSP a day of fermented food, to omit sugar—and to remember meat creates no alchemy, in my opinion.

Dr. Stephen Collins, a gastroenterologist at McMaster University is intrigued by the work of our gut feelings and how our intestinal bacteria influence our mood. He calls these bacteria "chemical factories" that affect the brain in two ways:

> Diet is one of the major influences on the metabolic activity of bacteria and if you now believe that these bacteria are in constant communication with the brain, then it's absolutely possible that food can alter your mood and your mental status, via the microbiota.[59]

# Antibiotics Benefits, Overuse & the Missing Microbes

*When I saw results of a meta-analysis out of Mount Sinai Hospital …
looking at over 7000 patients with IBD and identifying frequent antibiotic
use as one of the main risk factors in developing IBD, I knew people needed
to know this!*

*~ Dr. Chutkan*

## The War on Bacteria Is the War on Us!

The introduction of antibiotics as a key player in preventing disease came
with a huge learning curve of the side effects of antibiotic resistance and
the destruction of the microbiome diversity that occupy people's guts. This
is why I have seen people with IBD find it incredibly difficult to heal.

Most antibiotics used in the US are given to livestock—an indirect
transference to flesh eater. As antibiotics have been used in cases as a
protocol to rid the body of pathogens, it is worth noting that prebiotic and
probiotic therapy may render greater, life-sustaining results.

Antibiotics may be the A-bomb* that destroys our gut flora the
fastest (Dr. Axe). The multitude of antibiotics and chemicals in our food
supply along with pharmaceutical drugs that suppress our ability to easily
decipher what food makes us sick, may be prime factors in the world
epidemic of disease. Diets high in cultured and fermented food and drink,
along with plenty of fibre, have been known to help the microbiome do its
job effectively.

Studies on the overuse of antibiotics found that it's no surprise that
antibiotics directly affect mental health. "This is called antibiotic-induced

psychosis and usually these patients normalized their behaviour when you stop this antibiotic treatment."

In the largest study of its kind, antibiotic use in young people with Crohn's disease was found to worsen the imbalance of bacteria. The study took biopsies of 447 individuals with new diagnosis of Crohn's disease and 221 non-affected individuals. At multiple sites throughout the GI tract, the team found that patients with Crohn's had significant loss of beneficial microbes and an increase in pathogenic microbes.[60]

Dr. Zach Bush says he sees continued antibiotic-induced depression and anxiety at his M Clinic and his patients are never informed that anxiety risk goes up 17% after one course of antibiotic, 24% high risk of depression which will double after two courses.

In August 1928, Dr. Alexander Fleming left on vacation, arriving back in September to find his petri dishes inoculated with *staphylococcus* bacteria. As the story goes, something caught his eye as he was now tossing out the useless plates. He saw that the layers of billions of bacterial cells had grown wall to wall in the dish, but disappeared near the mould. The mould was identified as *Penicillium notatum* and the rest is so-called history. Fast forward into present day where antibiotic overuse has created enormous outbreaks as what is most commonly referred to as antibiotic resistance.[61]

***If fungus mold can kill bacteria, why can't they kill pathogens? Maybe that is why our bodies produce mould when we are not well.***

When we look at the short and long term negative effects of antibiotic use, such as skin rashes, nausea, diarrhea, candida, systemic yeast infection—and even death from antibiotic resistance—we must begin to explore the root cause. *Clostridium difficile (C. diff)* and other infections are easily spread from person to person through bacteria spores that are capable of living on surfaces for many days. It is estimated that up to 30,000 people a year in the USA alone die *of C.diff.*[62]

A routine course of action for a person with IBD is to be given a wide-spectrum antibiotics. When we look at bacterial overgrowth, which is most common in IBD and IBS, known as Small Intestine Bacterial Overgrowth (SIBO), antibiotics are often prescribed.

At this phase in my healing, affected by SIBO, my integrative medicine doctor put me on berberine, oil of oregano, and a multi-strain probiotic, which allowed my body to rid itself of the overpopulation of bacteria in my small intestines. The majority of bacteria in a healthy digestive tract should be in our large colon and not overgrown in our small intestine. This displacement makes a critical difference in our health.

*As cultures around the world become more 'Western,'*
*they lose bacteria species in their guts. At the same time, they*
*start having higher incidences of chronic illnesses connected*
*to the immune system, such as allergies, Crohn's disease,*
*autoimmune disorders, and multiple sclerosis.*

*~ **Martin Blaser***

**So the Big Questions:**

● What are we feeding our bacteria?

● May these commensal bacteria eventually assist us in overcoming peer pressure, herd mentality, neutralize pathogens?

● If most of our bacteria (90–99%) are good bacteria in a healthy host, then are we able to consider pre and probiotics, dietary shifts and meditation in place of medication?

## Meditation:

Sit quietly and feel into your belly. Imagine the good bacteria like PAC-MAN eating the pathogens. Imagine preparing and eating to feed your 100 trillion friends. Feel your belly breathing, settling and quieting your vagus nerves deep within.

## Gratitude:

I AM grateful for the microbes that keep me well and their ability to ward off disease.

I Am grateful for the power of daily healing and choice!

I AM ...

## Coming Homework:

Journal all your food for 3 months ... record how you feel 1–2 hours following each food choice.

Intend what you will change with this knowledge.

# PHOENIX

*Oh Phoenix Grandlad…*
*Coax me from this little screen*
*Of word upon word of a life we deem*

*As Aspen falls yellow splendour*
*Crunch beneath our feet*
*And throw her compost high to breathe…*

*We laugh into new biology!*
*In microbes across leaves*
*WE BREATHE*

*As wild rose and hips we forage, her leaves of auburn farewell*
*And snow geese trill from 'ahhh' so high*
*You lift your sweet little face to ponder*
*WE BREATHE*

*A breath of this biome, you bring me home!*
*We laugh*
*We breathe*
*Around and around*
*Never goodbye…*

# Chapter 11:

## The Microbiome -
## Early Beginnings,
## Resiliency, &
## Antibiotic Connection

*When I saw results of a meta-analysis out of Mount Sinai Hospital …*
*looking at over 7000 patients with IBD and identifying frequent antibiotic*
*use as one of the main risk factors in developing IBD,*
*I said, people need to know this!*

*~ Dr. Robynne Chutkan*

Enriching our microbiome;
a pet brings the diverse
outdoor microbes to us.
Let us begin a child's life
in reverence.

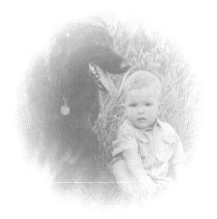

# Early Beginnings

Children are the living messages we send to a time we will not see, yet the research reveals almost 50% of our children will have a chronic disease of mindbody by 18 years of age. What is this earth our children are inheriting? Can we turn it around? Will we?

In the beginning, children were known to receive their first inoculation of bacteria through the vaginal canal upon entering this world, skin to skin, mouth to breast and lips from healthy parents who still interacted in a healthy environment.

This is where we see the beginning of a world out of harmony. Caesarean section surgery and bottle feeding may be necessary for parents unable to do natural birth and feeding, yet it is sometimes unnecessarily used too often for convenience and not always emergency—at the expense of a healthy diverse microbiome. I believe we, as a culture, are returning back to feeding our babies naturally when possible; and when not exploring breastmilk sharing, use natural formula as close to nature as possible. Other factors affecting early beginning are:

- Non-food stuff filling our schools, homes, chemical non-food

- Lack of contact with outdoors, and living nutrient-rich food and families preparing whole food together.

- Our convenience and fast-paced and overstimulated world

Breastfeeding is also a major contributor to the formation of a healthy microbiome. Healthy breast milk supports the maximum neurological growth. A breastfeeding baby begins life immediately with lipase and amylase nutrition. Pregnant breastfeeding mothers need adequate amounts of DHA, and the conversion of ALA to DHA is more optimal with proper levels of B3, B6, magnesium, zinc, and vitamins A, C, and E.

Oligosaccharides, which are plentiful in breast milk, promote the growth of Bifidobacterium and Lactobacillus, which assist in strengthening development and immunity.[70]

This was the case for myself when my mother was diagnosed with an aneurism when I was only ten days old. During this time, I was given watered down canned evaporated milk. As the story goes, I cried 24/7. My new normality throughout my early childhood was fluctuations of a distended, crampy abdomen—fluctuating between bouts of constipation and diarrhea. This was exasperated by the continual antibiotic prescriptions that I used for constant ear infections, which I later learned were due to my extreme allergies to sugar, processed food and dairy. There has always been a direct link to dairy allergies, loss of microbiota diversity and ear infections. This is the seeds for IBD and dis-ease, later in life for many.

Sheryl McCumsey, from *Pesticide Free Alberta*, and Zen Honeycutt, in *Moms Across America*, along with thousands of more trailblazing, advocating mother bears, teach the power of eating only organic and biodynamic food to heal allergies, learning disabilities, and more severe conditions, and are having great success.

The instinct to protect our children is strong, deep, and, old. I believe most mothers who have been given the correct information regarding the poison in our food supply, would protect their children from the tainted foods found in the supermarkets today.

# Early Childhood Exposure;
# Research of Significance

*We have realized that early life is a key window of vulnerability.*
*Young children have critical periods for their growth, and experiments*
*are showing that the loss of friendly gut bacteria at this early stage of*
*development is driving obesity. ... Ultimately, we seek to reverse the*
*damage seen around the world, including establishing strategies for*
*restoring the missing microbes... The antibiotic eliminates susceptible*
*microbes all over the body, along with the pathogen that usually is*
*present in one place. It is like a carpet bombing when*
*a laser-like strike is needed.*

*~ **Dr. Martin Blaser in Missing Microbes** [58]*

When looking at IBD and the connection with antibiotics, it is of value for us to consider a 2011 study, in which 577,627 children born in Denmark between 1995 and 2003 were followed. In this longitudinal study, 117 children developed IBD, 84% of which had received antibiotics compared to the healthy children who had received none. The investigators calculated that with each course of antibiotics there was an 18% increase in the development of CD. This is seven times greater risk of developing IBD than those who received no antibiotics.[58]

With breastfeeding *Bifidobacteria infantis* supplement—(a first strain often absent in C-section babies), my C-sectioned grandson's digestive issues were resolved.[58]

# Epigenetic, the Inner Child Diet, & Perfect Digestion

Epigenetics has discovered, through repeated scientific research, less than 10% of our diseases are created from hereditary factors. The two greatest influences in the first seven years of life are environment and how we perceive that environment. Dr. Bruce Lipton reminds us that in the first seven years we are walking around in a creative, theta-hypnotic state, and all our programming is based on our environment and how we perceive it. This becomes our unconscious and is usually what is running about 95% of the movie of our lives.

Our minds are incredible. I have witnessed this countless times through spiritual communities, at wellness and rejuvenation centres and within my own life—HOPE FLOATS.

So, in studying perfect digestion, our redemption comes from expanding and continually cultivating the consciousness we have access to. Our gut is often referred to as our second brain. HeartMath Institute research reveals that the heart has longer and stronger cellular memory than the brain. One thing is now certain, all three are communicating and deeply interwoven in a multidimensional matrix of our EarthGut from prebirth, into lifetimes and lovetimes made manifest. In the first few of years of life, the "domestication programming" as spoken of in *The Four Agreements*, isn't in place; so children often still belly breathe, choose fruit, mother's milk, and sleep over stimulants and restlessness. The documentation on sugar as an addictive substance is undeniable.

Many of us have something which keeps us tied in. So our awakened journey is compassionate, complex, yet simple. Knowledge is power. Knowing what was programmed around food and drink, and choosing to reprogram unhealthy choices can save precious lives.

I have witnessed continually that we can shift from the damage done in childhood by an environment which was unaware. Our mindbody is incredibly resilient, self-healing, and forgiving. Outdoor earth crawling, and organic live food may also correct this. Health is a gift.

Yet, finding self-care and love, and making both a priority in such an over-stimulating world is essential. Radical self-understanding is a must if we are to shift habits into more self-loving ones and reset our biology. Getting support, as I have extensively over the last few years, is the greatest gift you will give yourself. Our moment-to-moment choices matter, and we will only change when we cultivate peace, love and happy microbes!

## Meditation:

Bring yourself to an early memory of yourself , sometime around five years old. See if you can feel what you were feeling and what is going on for you. Keep breathing into that time and space as an adult coming to comfort the young you. Come close and hold the child. Give them the feeling of being deeply seen, loved, and protected NOW. Use this meditation whenever feeling overwhelmed and alone. Tell your child: "WE GOT THIS"!

## Gratitude:

I AM… Infinite
I AM… ageless
I AM WELL

## Coming Homework

Read Conscious Parenting

Join community parent and grandparent groups advocating for real food

# Whole

We touch beloved
Our skin and hearts entwined
Baby suckles on breast
Skin to skin
We smile and laugh
As we tickle in the grass

We run and play like fawns
Through the forest of damp moss and fungi
Exploring, curiosity of never-ending magnitude
We touch, hold hands, and embrace
Stretching like babies across the Universe
WHOLENESS!

Undrugged
Unplugged
My creativeness shines
Because I ate from the gardens instead of chemical factories
I played on Earth
And my fidgetiness just meant…
I was a free child who still understood the needs of big movement
And big joy
and I played endlessly in the rich and
sweet microbial abundant mystery

*Chapter 12:*

# *Individualizing your Diet: Supporting Life*

*And I said to my body softly "I want to be your friend." It took a long breath and replied, "I have been waiting for this my whole life."*

*Nayyirah Waheed*

*In the human body, homeostasis is maintained at every level through the precise orchestration of an infinite variety of biochemical reactions.*

*Wolcott*

## *Respecting Biochemical Individuality*

Individualizing one's diet is an incredibly complex yet simple diverse healing protocol. That being said, there is often the paradox that will withhold every truth: simplicity underlines everything complex. This is our beautiful plight home.

It is out of my scope to suggest one diet or one protocol for any individual. This is a journey one must take with an incredibly knowledgeable and compassionate integrative functional medicine team. But it is in my scope to tell you "You are Loved" and you being reconnected and here, right now, can really matter!

Everything that I share has been based on accumulated knowledge through practice; in-depth study with trial and error; a Masters degree in plant-based nutrition; and my love for people, earth mother and living beings!

YET, it has appeared across the board that when people omit the animal foods which are heavy in pathogenic bacteria, fear and suffering, they cleanse, detox and rest; heal their microbiome; get support in wellness, and have healthy love and connection. They discover absolutely everything matters in the moment-to-moment choices they make. They learn to listen to their gut intuition. The problem with this is an inflamed microbiome will send us mixed messages and have us craving food and drink that can continually set up a positive feedback loop with negative impacts.

I have never known any other illness that can give us direct messages quicker than when we work and listen to the messages of the gut. For example, when I began taking the supplement powder L-glutamine, I was able to feel my gut settle down quite quickly after only one dose. With *ION*Bione*, one week, and with bowel rest, the belly can soften within a day. With fasting, bowel rest, and mindbody rest in nature I healed quickly.

Individualizing your diet and learning to mediate the dynamic process of mindfulness with your ever-changing nutritional requirements may be one of the most conscious, creative ways into deep listening. Every meal a blessing, every food an opportunity for earth connection.

I see this process as a threefold, circular, dynamic process—we receive, redo and release, around and around. The process of conscious connection with food is written deep within our ancestral codes, both genetic genotyping and our epigenetic phenotyping.

Gabriel Cousens' food bible, *Conscious Eating*, is dedicated to deeply understanding food and its psychological impact. Exploring the psychosomatic process of food addiction is interesting and near to my heart. The roots of overstimulation and disconnect originated many years ago with the introduction of alcohol and drugs, such as sugar and caffeine, into many of our tribes, from utero onward. It was snuck in somehow much like excitotoxins, GMO/GE food of today, and over-medication.

- I suppose the question is: how do we make peace with ourselves so that food/drink are no longer unconscious seductions, and we are able to deeply listen to that quiet voice that directs us to the unique healing foods for our biochemistry, in that very moment?

- If we free our minds through meditation/prayer/service, releasing the obsession with self, will individualizing our diets become naturally balanced?

Waking up and looking around, it is clear, as a society, we are heavier animal and processed food eaters than ever before in history and… we are becoming more ill. One diet does not work for everyone. Our cells die, regenerate or rearrange with every breath, every ray of sunshine; therefore, so do the energy and ATP needs of our body electric. We are light returning to light. What we eat, drink and think either fuels the light or dims it. As important, is what we DO NOT eat, drink, think, and do.

Succeeding on a highly live-food, plant-based diet strengthens our intuition and guidance. Heavily cooked food does the opposite. We need our intuition and strength to navigate in these times of tipping point "progress."

There is definitely not one diet for everyone. Dr. Zach Bush says: "Let us stop arguing over macronutrients, when it all turns into the same thing, fuel for the mitochondria."

Yes, let us come back to food in its whole highly microbialized, mineralized state—whole, living nutrient, God-light, sun-food fuel!

**So possibly, the only question that remains:**
**Is this an anti-inflammatory food that restores my microbiome**
**and partakes in reciprocal love for Mother Earth?**

*In the second of surrender*
*The turning of the tides*
*In the waning and the waxing*
*I was here all along*
*Weaving your uniqueness, sweet one*
*Into the cosmos of all creation*

*And as this awakening unfolds*
*Simply breathe... weaving and marrying your infinite healing power*
*All this beauty which is YOU beloved!*
*All this delicious aliveness!*
*All of Earths' life weaving, tumbling to you*
*Into your unique and so precious*
*hallelujah heart*

## *Biochemical Individuality*

Every person has unique ability within their biochemical individuality for the following processes: assimilation; structural integrity; communication of neurotransmitters; circulation; defence and repair; ATP energy regulation; biotransformation and elimination; and, functional lifestyle with a unique bacteria diversity.

Therefore, the question may be asked; can we change and reset our biochemical individual reactions? For myself, after eating a low-glycemic diet, everything tastes sweet. After my microbiome adapted to eating plant based, I changed. Our biology can change quite quickly!

The best way to go about getting to know yourself is to fast for three days, then introduce one or two foods at a time and see what happens.

# Overstimulation Feeding Addiction

Our main balancing act is to avoid excess stimulation in all forms that take us away from intuition, listening and balance. Eating an anti-inflammatory alkaline diet clears your brain. When we are looking at "self-selection" in regard to food and drink, and one's ability to access "body wisdom" with regards to addiction, it appears there is a frequency, a resonance correlation, between nutrition and addiction. This is illustrated in biochemical individuality; furthermore, with respect to the ability to make wise food choices, it is clear that good nutrition is an important factor.

Sugar addiction has been found in extensive experiments involving small children being given a free choice of sugar in their diets that, when the children are adequately nourished with a diet containing the proteins, minerals, and vitamins that they need, they voluntarily eat less sugar. The documentary, *Fed Up*, depicts this well. It is evident that good nutrition promotes the wisdom of the body. Mice will work harder for a drink of sugar water than cocaine after being cocaine addicted. When I share this with my veterinarian daughter, she responds: "Good thing I am not a rat then, Mom." Humour, humility, and continuing the practice of respecting sovereignty, are a few of the gifts this quick-witted amazing woman has given me, while blessing me with motherhood.

Usually there are three stages of unravelling and redoing our diets to best support our spiritual evolution and divine dharma: **chaos, change and commitment.**

Chaos occurs as our body realigns when we clear past habits/addictions, healing the root causes and sorting through the clutter as we make "the next best choice."

As we begin to change, we are wise to implement at a peaceful, gentle, and forgiving pace. Dr. Cousens says moving from stage one (heavy animal and processed-food eating), to stage four (the way of the Essenes), may take years to do successfully and most addictions are gone after two years of a live-food diet.

In this time, focusing on what we have instead of what we are releasing, will be of great importance. There is this sweet balance that happens with many individuals when changing the epigenetic environment into a highly enzymatic, nutrition-rich terrain. The genetic "dispositions" towards obesity, alcoholism, and many disorders in this alkalized, energized terrain are unable to be made manifest. Cleansing allows us to reset our telomeres and intuition. Also, having a food journal is of great significance at this time. Journaling on how we feel one-two-three hours after a meal will provide information about how the food we are eating is metabolizing.

Meditation and prayer are significant at this time. Bodywork and all types of body awareness practices—such as yoga, zero-point, and walking—help me stay in the flow.

Commitment is sometimes the toughest part. The opponent will come out in full force and resistance and the saboteur will rear over and over. Hence, we have, within our divine heart, the ability to gratefully tap into something deeper.

When it comes to individualizing one's diet, "if some is good, more is not necessarily better." With highly nutritious food, we usually need to eat half as much food to receive maximum benefits in nutrition, spiritual deepening and anti-aging. This "less is more" is also true for supplementation. We must find our unique "sweet spot" and this will change as we build our nutritional reserves i.e., I may take three times the recommended dose of magnesium and have regular elimination whereas my daughter will have diarrhea.

# We Are in This Together

As individual as we are, there is one unlimited truth, service! All spiritual traditions know the ultimate truth, we are here to unite from a place of wholeness and sovereignty. Feeling good allows us to live our divine dharma, within community and family. It is difficult to serve when we are unwell.

We are always receiving spiritual guidance and inspiration when we open to receive. Great scriptures and great mystical teacher/poets such as Rumi or Hafiz help us solidify the connection between love and joy and how it relates to eating and living in the light. Allowing the impossible journey to manifest into awakened living thought, joy, and love is the hummingbird medicine.

Silence, fasting, meditation, and Kundalini awakening are easier to obtain with a high enzymatic, mineral-rich diet. This whole cosmic catastrophe would feel pointless without tapping into the matrix of a universal love and your reconciliation remembrance.

It is our birthright to be happy, healthy and free. We are not isolated beings and we couldn't be even if we tried.

**So what if our bottom line became this: We eat in a way that increases peace for all, keeping our eyes fixed on the golden path that has been laid out before us, receiving the presence through super food, super**

**strength and the super crystalline directive from DIVINE is about going deeper and deeper still.**

*Let us go deeper, go deeper, for if we do our spirits will
embrace and interweave and our spirits will be so glorious
not even God will be able to tell us apart.*

*Hafiz*

David Wolfe in *The Sun-Food Diet* says:

"When you eat raw plant food, your instincts become stronger, your intuition becomes more reliable and cleared, and decision making becomes effortless. You automatically tune into a different energy band of life."

As the awakening is unfolding; awareness is increasing and we may begin to connect our choices with the bigger picture; rapid extinction of species and fauna on our planet. Eating consciously means we eat for peace and protection for all, first and foremost, including ourselves. It means live-food clears us, so we may do our work—the work of AWAKENING. We are few, yet with strong God-conscious focus, our help is great.

Diets in general differ from this live-food cuisine. Many of us may miss the root cause of fatigue and disharmony such as: dehydration first and foremost; mineral/vitamin/enzyme deficiencies; nutritionally deficient foods; the connection of long-term impacts on heavy animal protein consumption; kidney depletion; acidity; global poison; and lack of joy, love, and creativity, in childhood, home and work life. Many diets are based on short-term gratification. Live-plant cuisine is built on very ancient healing truths from Pythagoras, Jesus, the Essenes, etc., and encompasses a continual evolution of refining the cuisine to entail new-truths, sacred gardens, eating food in its natural state. This maintained integrity, we bestowing in reverence gardens, forage lands, and our internal gardens holds the intestinal integrity in place.

Most people come to new truths when they are defeated and are done with the insanity—do the same thing over and over, which is harmful to oneself, knowing full well they will suffer at least somewhat from the choice. Resetting sabotage behaviour, can begin the activation of intuitive wisdom, cleansing into grace.

When we understand we are actually primarily spiritual being having a human experience, we begin anew—studying ourselves with greater reverence; blessing our need for heart connections; releasing unhealthy thought form—while cultivating creative purpose, habits, and healthy community. Intuition (deep listening) helps one fine tune these stages, as we release domestication and mental and animal slavery, fear and non-truth.

**We must be hungrier for health than pseudo-comfort patterning. We must be hungrier for health than all the stuff we buy that will never fill the hunger!**

Yes, food has equated comfort for many of us for many years. It is our most ancient cellular memory-olfactory, yet it is not wise to focus on the past, in light of the task at hand. Olfactory memories have special connotations of gathering and connection. Yet the nervous system resets itself after 20 minutes; therefore instead of grabbing something unhealthy, we can drink two glasses of water and eat a good fat/protein combo such as almonds or hemp hearts mixed with spirulina/chlorella. This decision will usually clear the cravings and the craving will pass if we stop focusing on the emotional food substance, used like a drug. Bringing movement into the equation always is a great assistant.

For many people it is finding, within a healthy community, a place to share real food and meals. This requires refining and detoxing everything many of us once knew as the correct way to exist and interact, on this forgiving little blue and green ball hurtling through space.

When the teacher appears and we have a deep commitment towards change and growth, if we are compassionate with the process of divine timing within ourselves, we can extend that "learn in order to give" as the teaching goes. This understanding is important for long-term change in our communities.

**A little piece of knowledge implemented may begin a person's journey towards freedom food. We gently plant seeds and continue to be watered and shone upon. We do the same for ourselves. There is nothing more powerful than a truth whose time has come to pass.**

The more we let go of the mycotoxic, non-food stuff, and live in our pH balance, we ignite our live bio-photonic body electric, while deepening our strength and guidance. The pH only has to drop to 6.9 before a person's brain begins to get hazy. Most people are much more acidic than that. Cancer, viruses/bacterial infections, arthritis and other diseases rarely exist in an alkaline system. Many minerals such as calcium, selenium and other essential minerals are leached from bones to balance the pH and begin the degeneration cycle. We are biochemical individuals in control of our ever-changing inner ecosystem. An alkalized life is a culture of self-love made manifest. This entails a culture of living waters and sun-food, whispering our ancient knowledge of our healed EarthGut, non-dualistic connection.

Often times us humans are motivated to change through pain and suffering. As a teacher once said to me: "Nothing tastes as good as feeling good feels!"

# Biogenetic Photonic Food Is for Every Individual

*"In essence, everything becomes transported into an electrical charge that interacts with the zero point mothership. The waves, or bio-photons, which are both particles and waves, are, in essence, energy communicators that transmit energy. The concept of non-locality, which essentially means that all subatomic particles are in contact with each other whether they are one mile apart or ten thousand miles apart, becomes the basis of intuition."*

*Dr. Gabriel Cousens.*

We tap into the ONENESS when we increase our micro-electrical potential within our body's cells. This takes place with highly cellular, metabolic electron food that is directly from the source (sunlight), mineralized soil, water and life. Our health depends on our ability to attract, store, and conduct solar energy that increase our bio-photon storage. Bio-photons are visual measures of the energy vibrancy in our food. A highly mineralized and solar enzymatic die can heal a mineral deficient society.

Dr. Szekely, great scholar of the Essenes, classified foods into four categories:

- Biogenetic—life generating (sprouts, seaweed etc.)
- Bioactive—life sustaining food (organic, live fruit, and vegetables)
- Biostatic—life slowing food (cooked organic food)
- Bioacidic—life destroying food (alcohol, processed food, etc.)

Live-food easily carries minerals into our body through ionic angstrom–size processes. Dr. Linus Pauling, winner of two Nobel prizes, said: "We can trace every sickness, every disease ultimately, to a mineral and nutrient deficient organism."

> *Minerals are the sparks of life. All body processes*
> *require minerals to activate enzymes."*
>
> **Mirabel Arizpe.**

In my Essene teachings I understood eating uncensored and from the earth, rather than from factories, is an ancient Essene practice. Many ascended masters such as Jesus and the Essenes knew this. Traditional yogis such as Rameen and the Sattva community, practice this. Raw plant food helps an average person become extraordinary, while obtaining superior health and unlocking many dormant powers. Plant-based veganic cuisine focuses on disrupting the compost button that may have turned on, deranging our biological terrain.

So we gather, collect strength, practice, meditate, and serve, while keeping our living and highly mineralized hearts shining light. We continue listening for the sound of pineal gland in the centre of our head and decalcifying the pineal gland through nutrition and iodine.

We continue gathering our sweetness from service, dharma and dream mastering. This is how we become successful on the highest super-foods available to us on the planet—we LIVE the truth in every breath and then the truth sets us free!

In research and personal experience, it is observed that CD flare-ups and increased gut inflammation occurred after many types of meals. When half of the meals were elemental diets relapse rates declined to 27%. When the study continued to a full elemental diet the remission rate over 1 year was 95.4%. The study indicated that Westernized diets cause dysbiosis in the gut microbiome. When beneficial bacteria and a semi-vegetarian diet (½ serving of fish once a week and ½ a serving of meat every second week was implemented) the relapse rate was 0% after 1 year and 8% after 2 years.[63]

For myself, in the acute stages of this disease, a three week supported detox, within a wellness centre, was a life-saving and life-changing experience. The one thing to consider, of paramount importance, is the Jarisch-Herxheimer Reaction—the increased symptoms that happen from the die-off effect of pathogenic bacteria.

The body is a self-healing organism by design, if we learn to get out of the way. It is quite amazing all bowel toxicity is gone and telomeres reset after only seven days of a green juice cleanse. Mindbodies given proper love and respect within the natural laws heal. We experience this when we cut ourselves, break a bone or heart, time heals and a favourable environment helps us heal quicker.

Sweet Creator and Mother Earth hold every herb, seed and fruit bearing medicine necessary for health and regeneration; as in Genesis 1:29. Exploring health and regeneration through peace, love, and microbes gives us a wider view.

Love has always begun with us. Love has no bottom. Love is one place we can place our trust, knowing the bottom will never fall out if we are deeply centred in love rather than fear. In these times of extreme change, fear will throw us off our centre very quickly.

In that sweet surrendered place, we are able to hold the light within, for another: non-causal love that emits without expectation. We naturally move into the rhythm of natural laws, where our sensitivity to all life becomes acute and poisons in all forms, fall away. Food, as Dr. Gabriel

Cousens inerates is "our love note from God" and is available in the soil, the trees the plants the microbes—available for us all.

Our microbiome is so very sensitive to stress and toxins. Gratitude in every interaction, is the lovely antidote to stress.

## Meditation:

Sit quietly and breathe. Allow yourself to feel the unique cellular matrix you are. Smile into every organ-one by one, cultivating gratitude for each. Stay here as long as you wish.

## Gratitude:

I AM grateful for my unique gifts I bring the world.

I AM grateful I live in a way that supports my unique ever-changing-nutrition-requirements, while supporting the health of the planet.

I AM…

## Coming Homework:

Make a committed nutrition plan for the next month which
includes highly hydrating and nutrition-packed food.
Pay attention to how you feel.

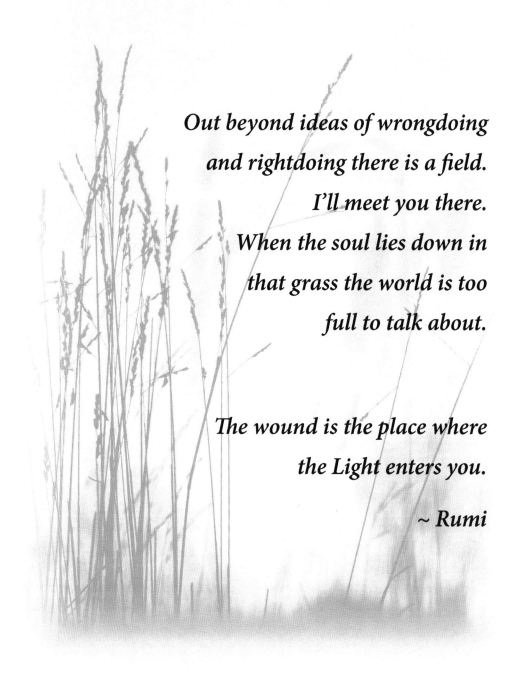

*Out beyond ideas of wrongdoing*
*and rightdoing there is a field.*
*I'll meet you there.*
*When the soul lies down in*
*that grass the world is too*
*full to talk about.*

*The wound is the place where*
*the Light enters you.*

*~ Rumi*

# Chapter 13:

## Aging well, Happy & on Purpose: We - The Synthesis of Heaven and Earth

*We would be wise to adopt the pace of nature"*

*~ Emerson*

I sink into Mother Earth and contemplate how the deep connection, respect and nurturing of her microbial mystery is a sevenfold sacred peace made manifest. I realize that most diseases are modern day afflictions due to lifestyle choices we may or may not know about, and systemic stress and world poisoning. Most degenerative diseases have become our modern day dilemmas, as we moved away from root cause health care to symptomatic treatments rooted in only pharmacology. Health towards regeneration looks at the root cause of most disease—stress, toxicity, acidity, loneliness, toxicity, and inflammation, which are at epidemic proportions.

Most of us have seen people fight an illness or endure extreme stress and observe, "it is like they aged overnight." Well, they have, both chronologically which speaks to years counted from birth and biologically. We live in a pseudo-young-hungry society: poisoning injections, liposuction, surgery, toxic topicals, along with well-formulated anti-aging EVERYTHING.

In order to thrive, our ability to repair must be at greater rate then the injury our body withstands - the young repair and regenerate stem cells much faster. Sadly, many youth of today are not repairing quickly anymore. Even some young babies are unable to repair and generate enough B cell action to produce the magnitude of antigens needed to fight toxic overload and leaking gut loses track of how to fight autoimmune dysregulation. Our villi lymph can produce 100 million B cells per day when given a favourable terrain.

Let us turn this around fast.

**The top three scientifically validated variables for healthy longevity are:**

◊ Whole food plant-based nutrition

◊ Being adaptive to reduce stress load in these precarious times, (meditation and healing our EarthGut is the balm).

◊ Love and connection

# *The Origin of Degeneration: Coming Home*

When we switch to eating light food, the aperture on the end of our cells are able to uptake or provide the redox electron charge to communicate with each other.

I was recently listening to three women in my GI doctor's waiting room speaking of severe allergic reactions they were having to Remicade (an autoimmune suppressant drug) that they were on for Crohn's and Colitis. One of the women said she had been hospitalized for the first time since her disease began. I experienced the same thing, ten years previous when I began this medication. I did a twelve-day, whole-body fast and came clean. Remicade, just one of the many pharmaceutical immunosuppressants used in inflammatory disease management, has allowed people to go into remission. For some individuals, suppression of symptoms may only last two years or less and risk the side effect "may cause cancer."

In understanding Maslow's hierarchy of needs, we find physiological needs are at the bottom and self-actualization is at the top as each of us move into being a creative, morally responsible, problem-solving person. We see a contrast to how many people are barely just getting by today. In a culture of dis-eased and overfed and undernourished people; we are now given the opportunity on this beautiful planet to awaken!

Cancer, diabetes, heart disease and autoimmune disease cannot be separated from society's big shoulder shrug, inject and reject the obvious. Poison and slavery can only go in one direction—down. Outsourcing our food and imprisoning animals is creating a karmic refund of disease.

Even if we do not believe in karma, we would be very wise to not overlook the obvious. The only way we can continue to destroy our ecology, is when we have completely lost touch with good. We are at the forefront of becoming solarly charged. It is our personal responsibility to understand the food and pharmaceutical industries' successful marketing campaigns. Information has been withheld while we create addicted and dependent people.

Separation is as dangerous for our health, as reclaiming deep connection is dangerous to big agriculture chemical companies and big pharma investors.

Junk food manufacturing and consumption is one of our most profound examples of cultural forgetting; electron lovers' farm to our tables of living food, love, and laughter.

If our point of power is our mouth, as stated by the father of Macrobiotics, Michio Kushi, then junk food represents a complete loss of cultural power. Choices are actually taken away when we remove vigour, peace, and our ability to see, feel and walk, as many diseases end in. Elevated blood sugar and insulin resistance adversely affects every disorder. Reclaiming our power is wisely choosing what goes in and out of our mouths.

Adapted from: Biology Basecamp by Zach Bush, MD.

| Biome Imbalance - Leaking Gut- Leaky Brain Inflammation Cascade through Lifespan: | |
| --- | --- |
| YEARS | DIS-EASE |
| 0 - 10 | Colic, ear infections |
| 10 - 20 | Strep, ear infections, depression |
| 20 - 30 | Depression, sleep disorders |
| 20 - 40 | Insulin resistance, infertility, autoimmunity |
| 40 - 60 | Autoimmunity, opportunistic infections, vascular disease, cancer |
| 60 - 70 | Dementia.[1] |

**Remembering… the Culture of Life**

*Raw plant foods, medicinal herbs, laughter, bliss, joy,*
*and unconditional love all exist in the same frequency range.*
*The tuning into this frequency raises the overall vibration*
*in a lower frequency range, such as fear, pain, doubt, cancer,*
*ugliness, depression, toxins, and so on, to eventually percolate*
*out and be ejected from the body.*
*This process is known as 'detoxification."*

*David Wolfe*

Radical acceptance of one's body is essential when we realize that over 80% of young females do not like their bodies. This is a huge representation of superficial culture of death programming. The feminine energy will be what allows us to reconnect and want to partake in coming home.

Buddha said everything begins and ends with thought. Peace with the mind is the beginning of remembering. Whenever I do body work with someone I always begin with breath-work. I can detect when they begin to think again when their body begins to tense. This is a profound example of how seldom our thoughts promote peace.

We must find a way to love ourselves enough to make the changes that support us. Most if not all degenerative disease have a digestive link. It would be wise for us to continue connecting these dots.

# *Eating Sugar, Animal Products and Grain*

When the villi on the small intestines are compromised, grain and heavy meat usually rots in the gut. I heard two men speaking over dinner this year how terrible their flatulence smells if they eat red meat.

This is worthy of mention again! Much research regarding the effects of grains on inflammation, (especially conventional gluten grains), suggests we omit them for well-being.

Sugar is a disaccharide double sugar, indigestible in a gut with flattened and damaged intestinal villi. Most fast food contains toxic trans fats, sugar, and gluten. This life of convenience is "crimes against wisdom," as Gabriel Cousens reiterates. Rameen Peyrow says he is unable to get over how seemingly intelligent people treat their body-temple.

## *Calorie Restriction & Exercise =Longevity*

When we do a deep hydration protocol and stop eating we turn on all the anti-aging genes and give the body a chance to catch up in the job of ridding the body of toxins.

Deep cellular hydration is the first protocol. Calorie restriction turns on the anti-aging, anti-inflammatory, antioxidant, and anticancer genes, as research indicates.

In conscious eating we become aware that a live-food organic diet allows us to eat half the amount of calories for satiation because cooked food coagulates 50% of the protein, and destroys 70% of the nutrients and 95% of the phytonutrients.

The China Study by Colin Campbell also shows the higher the plant-based food eaten, the less amount of disease. Many other scientist doctors, such as Gabriel Cousens, have proven the same. Research regarding "less is more" is coming from every direction in medicine as long as the less is nutrition-dense.

# Neurogenesis

"Neuro" meaning brain and "genesis" new beginning—the brain is known now as plastic and amiable, able to revisit a new beginning. This means we can grow new brain cells at any time, rewire into healthier habits and recreate a new "biology of belief," as Dr. Bruce Lipton teaches in his book of the same name. This is the study of neuroplasticity and resetting epigenetic programming at any age.

Let us rewire for health and peace. Plant medicine is our way home. David Crowe, master herbalist, with whom I have had the honour to study with, posed a very interesting question in his book, *In Search of the Medicine Buddha:*

"How and why do you want to grow old? Is it just to collect more entertaining experiences at the expense of the earth or is it to turn yourself and the planet around."

# Overstimulation as a Coping Strategy:

I have studied nutritional healing for two decades and have had enough long-term intervals of a symptom-free bowel, brain, and body to know what food and drinks to avoid. Yet, I am still get swayed on occasion. Keeping our face to the sun and our diet pure helps us create wiser choices.

Often, we discover that anything the body is sensitive or allergic to, will rob our health, and destroy our microbiome and our joy. An overstimulated body is the metabolism's way of speeding up, to rid the body of poison. I was recently in line at a grocery store. A little child in a shopping cart next to me was having a crying tantrum. Within a minute, I realized what it was about, when his mother gave him the box of Smarties he was screaming for. When Eric Clapton was asked where he believed his cocaine addiction began, he said, "Sugar." The same place in the brain lights up for sugar as it does for cocaine and heroin. Sugar and processed-food products are known to be good gut annihilators, blood sugar elevator, and can speed up degeneration. Sugar turns on advanced glycation end-product (AGE).

When did we become addicted to the feelings of overstimulation? Most likely, for many of us, it was in childhood beginning with the white sugar, white flour and chaotic, unsettled hearts. Many sensitive children adapted to a less than sensitive protective environment. Stimulation may have felt like the closest energetic match and soon became a "negative pair bonding."

It appears the abnormal has become normal. So here we are in a high-fashioned, paper-cup society of stimulant addicts, "business as usual" and it all seems "normal." Antidote? Get outside, play, look around, run through the trees, lay under a tree, become one with an arborist, play in living waters, be a child, let yourself be held and safely cared for—by yourself and another.

## *Gut Inflammation & Depression:*

*Not only can impairments in your microbiome promote neurological diseases, it can also have a powerful impact on your general mood. Depression is increasingly starting to be viewed as a symptom of poor gut health, and therein may lie the real cure as well.*

*Dr. Perlmutter in* Brain Maker

**Will it be considered a malpractice in the future to diagnose a mental disorder without first evaluating the integrity of the gut microbiome?**

Knowing the deep connection between the gut and the brain, we may conclude that everything that destroys our microbiome destroys our brain and our inherited right for joy, wise decisions and liberation.

Professor Bernstein at the Department of Gastroenterology at University of Manitoba discovered that mood disorders always precede gut problems. He found that having bacteria in your bowel triggers an immune response that also impacts brain function. "By manipulating the bugs in the bowel, one may be able to improve mood disorders."[64]

The vagus nerve that connects the brain to the digestive and immune system, and the heart is enriched with beneficial bacteria. Now mental illnesses and mood are being looked at through a microbial lens. Healthy fecal microbiota transplants into anxious mice have a dramatic calming effect, after only one transplant.

Many people with IBD get depressed. This is well-documented in the medical community. The connection is clear.

Given the ability of the gut microbiota to influence serotonin and its precursor tryptophan, and also to regulate the stress response, to grow younger biologically must include first and foremost a diet rich in microbiome builders, pre and probiotic whole foods while omitting all microbiome killers as spoken of throughout. The mindbody knows what to do and all we must do is get out of its way, and allow peace, love and healing microbes access in to re-groove our brains into healthy new synapses.

# *Tree of Life & Tree of Dis-Ease Exercise*

Draw your tree of life. Some people also find it useful to draw their tree of disease.In the roots of your ill tree, write about toxins and inflammatory thoughts which have been put into habitual actions into your life, which keep your "trunk" acidic and thirsty. How has the toxicity branched out into one of the various inflammatory / autoimmune diseases?

Now, draw your tree of life and the joy in your alkaline trunk and photosynthesized branches. Let us see disorders and diseases as just that, a deep disconnect from the order of nature's law and ease, from the nourishing roots up! See nature's laws of harmony and ease returning to your microbial-rich earth, feeding the roots with highly mineralized organic matter, resetting the pH balance and sending off new happy shoots into the heavens. Uproot deep roots of disease and death through changing some less-than-desirable habits that are deeply entwined into old patterns. Live perseverance and self-love, connecting with the oneness.

Once we dig up the dying roots and bury them deep into new soil, we must feed the soil with microbes and sea minerals. Welcome home, Earthling! This journey will smell sweet like a newborn alkaline baby; taste sweeter than ever before, and feel better than we could have ever imagined. A healthy Tree of Life allows us to reset regret. This is our freedom food. Colour your tree.

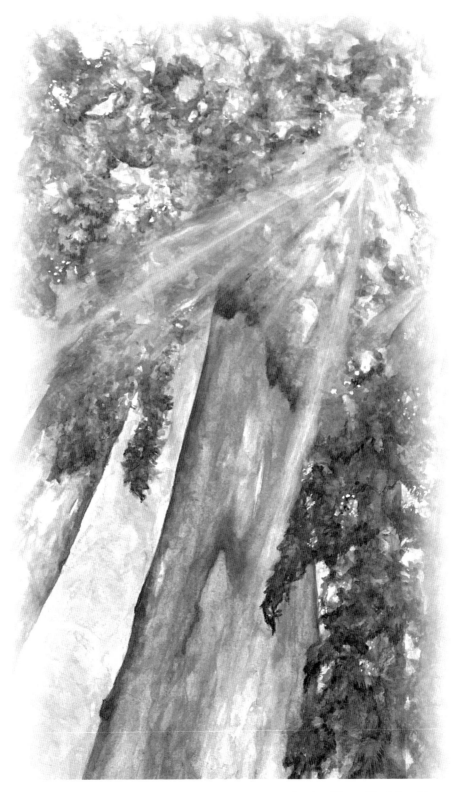

## Story:

I lived with IBD for a few years and seen my body waste rapidly before my eyes! Inflammation ages us fast! It was astonishing to feel the gut/brain connection, as I went from an optimistic go-getter to a very sad being. I have compassionately witnessed this in many others.

I have also experienced the incredible regenerative powers of the body, in both my recovery of bowel disease and a shattered right leg, after which I was told I may never walk again without a cane. An amazing surgeon saved my leg, as they told me amputation, due to extreme damage, was probable. Surgery was successful. I rested for three months, meditated and experienced a deep surrender in just staying put. I chlorophyll-enriched my way through heart-green chakra litres of fresh organic juice, salads, super-foods, and rest. Many of my days were one solid meditation. I have little scar tissue and am fully alive and healed, hardware removed.

Actions we choose in every moment matter. Conventional and commercial Roundup ready food destroys our healthy floras as do some pharmaceuticals. Let us remember the Hippocratic Oath, "First do no harm." This oath is also the oath of the Essenes, integrative physicians and trailblazing wellness seekers/teachers.

In Ayurveda medicine, disease begins with accumulation and stagnation. In Chinese medicine disease has two root causes: deficiency and excess—often a deficiency in minerals, hydration, whole plant foods, exercise, purpose and peace; an excess of acids, toxins and inflammation, accumulated emotional residue, and a diseased inner terrain.

Many people put ALL their faith in the allopathic doctors, who are pharmaceutically trained, not nutritionally trained. Let us look at integrative approaches.

# Story:

Just recently, I was speaking with a client who shared her excitement of visiting a remote village in Costa Rica. She said as soon as she stepped off the boat from a ride of 1.5 hours down a canal, she was in a rich forest surrounded by water, life, monkeys, etc. and she instantly felt a relaxation she had not felt before. Perhaps, just perhaps, the ancients and microbial minions were reminding her of a thriving ecosystem of forgotten times, a fulvic ancient soil diversity alive!

When we begin the journey to thrive, instead of simply survive, we honour and build living soil that, in turn, shows up in our inner eco-garden—from wilted to wondrous. When we make the commitment to listen to our gut instincts, we may reclaim our birthright for peace, successfully arresting inflammation, myotoxicity, and disease.

The light is upon us. We can study the mountains of information at our fingertips and know more than our doctor about mindbody nutrition in a few days. Seeds of deception are being illuminated. The war on bacteria questioned. A food revolution is taking place at every bend, calling us back home to our thriving biology and our honoured place at our table.

## Meditation:

Breath in your Divine and out your suffering, as in the Buddhist practice of Tonglen: every breath in new life, and every breath out a mini death. Ask to be given the intuition food, supplementation and sweet nectar of life, which will give you experience, strength and hope. Be with this. Journal the messages

## Gratitude:

I AM grateful I can clear my mind and just breathe.

I AM grateful the truth of wellness is coming my way.

I AM…

I AM THAT WHICH I AM…

## Coming Homework

What will you write down as a focused intention for the next seven days; to turn off degeneration and build a new mindbody?

We can create a new body in a year, begin to create a new mindbody in 24 hours! This is a biological truth. What are you feeding your beloved self today—love or not?

*When you ingest prebiotic fiber,*
*the fermentation that takes place*
*in your gut helps with water and*
*electrolyte reabsorption and produces*
*short-chain fatty acids (SCFAs)*
*which help maintain the lining of the bowel.*
*Water soluble fiber is fermented*
*well by your gut microbiota.*

*~ Dr. Challa*

# Chapter 14:

## *Repair and Maintenance of a Healthy Mindbody Microbiome/Pre- & Probiotics Supplementation*

*Lactobacillus competes with potential pathogens for receptor sites at the mucosa cell surface of the intestines and proposes a treatment strategy of "eco-immunonutrition."*

**Sandor Katz in Wild Fermentation** [65]

Going back to being earth-people now, we collect our missing microbial melody! First supplement will always be Mother Nature's diversity!

In my journey through IBS and IBD, I have used my own body as an experimental lab. The most challenging part of this healing opportunity has been to feel as though I'm doing everything that I know how to do, and then to still get recurrence of severe symptoms. It was only when I realized that in whole-person healing, even one piece of the medicine wheel out of balance or missing will prevent the body from healing. For example: adding just one allergen to the equation can trigger hyper-permeability and start a landslide of symptoms, even when I was doing absolutely everything else "perfectly." Another example could be not addressing the mindbody-heart-stress connection. Emotional stress and mental dis-ease can linger and can cause physical symptoms, as sure as any other factor.

## 3 P's of a Healthy Microbiome & 33 Gems of Mastery

### Protect

Protect your microbiome so that you may always be healthy and able to neutralize and destroy harmful microbes.

Protect your heart with a supportive community, radical self-love, and meaningful service.

Protect your brain with brain nutrition, meditation and rewiring for self-empowering healing.

Build your microbiome, otherwise known as your largest immunity. When in harmony, it can play an instrumental role in how our body functions. Protect and rebuild it!

### Persevere

We are walking conduits between heaven and earth. Find the way of natural hygiene eating, of living loving biome diversity, while allowing life to resonate and awaken the inner physician.

When we honour readiness and continue moving in the right direction, even if we have had to reset regret more times than we can count, we keep getting up. As in the words of poet Rumi, " It doesn't matter if you've broken your vows a thousand times or more … come come whoever you are, wanderer, worshipper lover of leaving!"

## Praise

Praising the gifts you've been given and always honouring that you are a divine spark of God, come home to your temple, caring for your body, mind and spirit in the sacrament. Build prana, build gardens and feeding your inner ecosystem so you may continue to remember your hallelujah heart.

## 33 Gems Towards Health Mastery Review

*The variation of the microbial diversity is based on many internal and external factors, such as:*

1. Diet of mind
2. Diet of food & drink—must be ORGANIC/VEGANIC/ BIODYNAMIC
3. Local real organic food gardens
4. Mode of birth . Natural childbirth
5. Ancestry & geographical location
6. Chemical and radiation influences
7. Hygiene—of body mind and spirit and over-sterile environments
8. Environmental factors and water source
9. Food supply and source
10. Activity level
11. Connection and gratitude gathered

## Beneficial bacteria, otherwise called probiotics assist in:

1. Healing systemic inflammation, leaky gut & disease causing bacteria
2. Produce vitamins, minerals and amino acids
3. Increase neurotransmitter activity, such as increasing serotonin (up to 90% of serotonin and 50% of dopamine is made in the gut)
4. Beneficial bacteria are the great toxin eliminators

5. Commensal bacteria known to elevate mood, and assist in bringing mental health into balance
6. Eliminate allergens
7. Modulate immune responses
8. Allow the body to find a healthy weight set-point
9. Protect from intestinal hyper-permeability
10. Help awaken and light us up
11. Protect systemically from degeneration and inflammation

## Health depends on:

1. Restoring gut integrity and probiotics ability to take hold
2. Prebiotics from earth-loved vegetables and fruit
3. Resident microbiota-early beginnings
4. Nutrients and vitamins
5. Hydration
6. Detoxification of mindbody
7. Whole-person health and allowing clarity to conduit the divine
8. Deficiency balancing with allergens removed
9. Deep connection: body heart mind and beyond
10. Quieting mindful practices, deep stress and anxiety avoidance—in all forms
11. Avoiding GMO/GE food and glyphosate, toxic food and drink

## The Four R's of Functional Medicine Plus One

**1.REMOVE:**

It has become well known that there will be nothing—no supplement, no probiotic, no amount of mindbody integration that will be able to keep the intestinal integrity in place without removing ALL sensitivity foods, chemicals, glyphosate and allergens.

This bowel lining can be likened to semipermeable "cheesecloth"—optimally tightly woven and protected by the mucosa barrier. Again, the bowel lining regenerates every 72 hours! This is quite amazing when you think of what an incredible self-healing organism the body is. Yet, this new lining is sensitive and is very easy to disturb.

During this regeneration time of the mucosa lining, liquid diets that eliminate large amounts of fibre are usually crucial. This may include a water, green juice, smoothie and/or elemental diet fast. It cannot be overemphasized that understanding the critical importance of removing allergenic food; grains which are high in mycotoxicity and disaccharide and difficult to digest, and food such as meat, gluten, eggs, and dairy—are crucial at this time. "This time" may mean a lifetime if someone is to continue to remain in remission medication-free.

Recent research has indicated that the majority of people suffering from an autoimmune disease and/or depression have intestinal hyper-permeability. For example: when people who report themselves as "not allergic: to gluten are tested, intestinal hyper-permeability increases for an hour, and in people who are truly allergic, for at least four hours. When we understand that the majority of people who are not on a gluten-free diet often have some form of gluten several times throughout their day, it would be wise to understand the increased toxic load that is damaging the mucosa lining and allowing the "cheesecloth" to open, creating systemic inflammatory damage and an incredible amount of toxins to flow into the bloodstream.

Native herbs and supplements have been used to remove the harmful bacteria quickly:

- Wormwood
- Berberine

- Oil of oregano
- Caprylic acid [72]

*Following is a summary of some of the teachings of* The Culture of Life:

- Remove chemical/pesticide/herbicide and GMOs from our topsoil
- And our plates: remove all toxic trigger foods that are not correct for our biochemical individuality.
- Eliminate all negative thoughts towards ourselves and others that consume us and our planet.
- Eliminate using our bodies and our earth as a dumping ground.
- Eliminate, as much as, possible electromagnetic pollutions, heavy-handed practices, and heavy hearts.
- Eliminate everything that enslaves all sentient beings and does not feed our good bacteria. Possibly eliminate prebiotic food for a short time in the early healing times so we do not feed SIBO.

## 2. REPLACE

Consider what our inner and outer ecology needs to survive and repair. Asking some questions:

- What is the exact food that are both pre and probiotic, that work for my individual biochemistry?

- What plants grow best in the soil?

- What do I need and what do I need to eliminate in order to be well; where is the sweet spot the exact amount of nutrition and water to receive maximum health (too much of a good thing becomes poison)?

- What would I be feeling if I wasn't eating?

## 3. RE-INOCULATE

Grow food in healthy living soil, consume Effective Microorganisms, eat cultured food re-inoculate by grounding barefoot to the earth, consume probiotics and take digestive enzymes / sauerkraut with meals, and eat veganic, raw, and close to nature. In addition to consuming soil-enriched food and fulvic and humic acid, repopulate with beneficial bacteria strains that build and repair.

After pathogens are gone, prebiotic foods containing either inulin or arabinogalactans may help the body build good flora: foods such as asparagus, carrots, garlic, artichoke, leeks, onions, radishes, jicama, and tomatoes.[34]

## 4. RESTORE/REPAIR

This healing of the bowel lining begins to happen quickly if toxic food is eliminated.

As we restore the gut's microbiome, the following supplements have been used to regenerate: Fulvic acid and trace minerals such as in Exalt by Promedics, zinc; vitamin C; L-glutamine; aloe vera; quercetin; slippery elm; deglycerized licorice (DGL); marshmallow root and gamma oryzanol, *ION\*Bione* by Biomic Science Lab LLC, CBD, and probiotics in nature and food mostly.

It may only take two days of eating well for the microbiome to begin to change composition and sugar cravings begin subsiding.

## 5. RECONNECT

Like beautiful
granddaughter Emerlee

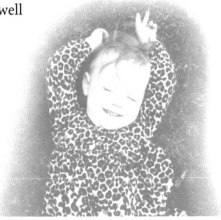

# *Probiotics*

Probiotics, live multi-strain commensal bacteria means "for life"; prebiotics are the food that feed the probiotics and the microbiome bacteria. It is important to understand prebiotics feed pathogens also. A protocol to remove pathogens is important. Many probiotics are no longer alive; be wise.

Commensal bacteria adhere to the mucosa wall preventing hyper-permeability created by pathogenic bacteria. Commensal bacteria produce antimicrobial substances that help protect against the environment of pathogenic bacteria. Probiotics overused can build mono cultures in the gut and although targeted probiotics for short time may be helpful, diversity is the key.

In understanding that the majority of our immune system is in our gut, it is relevant to explore how probiotics have worked in immunomodulation of such issues such as IBD. It appears that probiotics may affect immune system a threefold manner.

1. Production of immunoglobulin A (IgA)—big word but simply—proteins that recognize foreign invaders which probiotics have been shown to increase production when needed and neutralize.
2. Decrease of inflammatory mediators.
3. Decrease antibodies that are allergy-specific to allow the body to fight irritating external substances, such as pollen and animal dander.

In the work of many functional doctors, it is understood that in a mucosa compromised gut, the host may need to begin building up tolerance or real organic earth food that come with the highest resonance of beneficial bacteria.

"It is possible that the products of the commensal flora promote inflammation in the presence of an impaired mucosa barrier or injury to the mucosa… These results indicate that, in health, there is tolerance to autologous [your own] but not allogeneic [foreign source] intestinal flora, and tolerance is lost during inflammation. Evidence also exists that animals are tolerant to their own flora in health but not after colitis develops."

~ Claudio Fiocchi [67]

# *Prebiotics*

Prebiotics are understood as dietary fibre that provide nutrition for probiotics. The understanding of this interrelationship has only been explored since 1995.

Dr. Challa names three criteria that qualify a substance as a prebiotic[66]:

1. Resistant to gastric acidity not digestible by host
2. Able to be fermented by the gut microbiota
3. Stimulate growth and activity of the gut microbiota that contributes to your health and well-being

# *Researched Gut Restoration Probiotic Brands*

The probiotic synergist I have worked with over the last few years is Effective Microorganisms. I discovered it from biologist John Phillips at the Tree Of Life during a 30-day intensive when the stress of study, heat and being away created a flare up. One day using EM1 probiotic and my bowels settled. I have never had an experience such as this with any probiotic. VSL3 in the hospitals helped slow down loose stools but not huge effects, Natren proved some greater results, but now the medicine is ION*Bione is my intermittent combo with EM.

RESEARCHED AND TESTED Gut Support

**ION\*BIOME**

A unique & proprietary blend of natural ancient soil extracts that works to fortify your gut membrane & optimize your gut-brain connection.

**EXALT** by Promedics Canada

Helps heal the gut and has been effective for my gut and my people as well.

**EM 1 PROBIOTIC**

Here is what nature farmer biologist John Phillips says EM:

> EM is much much more than just a synergist! EM is, first of all, a probiotic common to healthy soil, plants, animals and humans. It is the unifying field of the biome. EM is a rich source of enzymes antioxidants and organic digestive acids that aid healthy digestion and prevent purturfaction. EM promotes fermentation under anaerobic or low oxygen conditions. EM stimulates the growth of helpful microbes which surround and neutralize pathogenic microbes." [16]

Biome Science's lab has found, through divine grace, the antidote in the ancient earth fossil terrahydrite that will strengthen and protect against even ridiculous glyphosate exposure. This team has researched that all 30-50 tight junctions are repaired in the light of terrahydrite. I know promoting another in the marketing realms are supposed to be the death of us, but people, it is too late, much too late to be politically correct in the "my piece of pie first" in this rapidly depleting planet. I am just here to give you the best I have deemed through endless study and money well spent in healing myself from death's door, a Masters degree in Live food Spiritual Nutrition specializing in the microbiome and... I deeply care enough to not care! So here I go promoting what heals.

- **NATREN** (most recommended by Jini Patel and well researched). There is a theory that saccharomyces—the soil based probiotic—will compete with other strains so they isolate probiotics[3]

- **GARDEN OF LIFE and PRIMAL DEFENSE** (Jordan Rubin) Garden of Life founder Jordan Rubin, who has healed a near-death encounter with Crohn's at the age of 19, he gives us "seven" secrets to healing the gut which he shares in soil based probiotics:

There are new products coming on the market daily, and some offer relief such as *Living Alchemy's* "prolife" supplement I have been testing. Yet, as mentioned throughout, a wise option is changing ones food source, first and foremost, to support gut health.

### Best Probiotics Is Nature's Wonderland & Establishing Health Flora Through Love Food.

*Bacillus subtilis* – works in the small intestines. Nato is the best source. It has the ability to break down hydrocarbons and create short-chain fatty acids

*Bacillus clausii* – amazing for the lungs. Helps build oxygen

*Bacillus coagulans* – for large intestines

*Saccharomyces boulardii* – for skin

*Lactobacillus plantarum* – for digestion, assimilation and the absorption of food in the gut. in abundance in sauerkraut

*Turkey Tail Mushroom* – an amazing prebiotic booster

Fermented herbs such as astragalus, ginger, and turmeric[68]

Note: one probiotic cell in the right environment in the gut doubles every 20 minutes. When our microbiota is stressed we have poor nutrition absorption, weight gain, diabetes, autoimmune disease, IBD, brain fog, and cancer. Overdosing on single strains may not be the answer long-term … diversity naturally has always led us home.

# How Do Strain Diversities Work?
# Not Necessarily Talking About a Bottle,
# But EarthGut Probiotics from Real Food.

Diversities of strains have different constructive use when improving gut health. The three main strains are divided into categories relating to their function:

## 1. *Lactobacillus* Species

The most common bacteria strain in the gut—predominantly resides in the small intestine or the upper gastrointestinal tract where a vast majority of your immune cells reside. They produce lactase and lactic acid via the fermentation of carbohydrates. *Lactobacillus* combats the growth of toxic microorganisms via the production of lactic acid and also functions in the absorption of iron, calcium, and magnesium.

- *L. acidophilus*: aids in optimal functioning
- *L. salivarius*: aids in optimizing nutrient absorption, disposing of waste and producing detoxifying enzymes which form on the mucosa layer of the intestinal wall
- *L. rhamnosus*: boosts the body's immune responses—increasing the level of the body's ability to circulate antibodies
- *L. plantarum* (found in sauerkraut, kimchi): beneficial strain which eradicates colonies of *E. coli* in gut. Has been found to be deficient and even almost extinct in many people's microbiomes—hence the power of sauerkraut!

## 2. *Bifidobacterium* Species

The second most important group of bacteria strains reside in the large intestine or the lower bowel, which is another critical location associated with health. They line the walls of the colon and act as a barrier to pathogenic microbes. In the ideology of IBD many people are missing this species. *Bifidobacteria* have also been known to prevent tumours in the large intestine by consuming the enzymes that contribute to the formation of tumours.[69]

## 3. Bacillus Species

Is the most resilient gut microflora—resisting the highly acid environment of our stomach.

### PREBIOTICS:
- Arabinogalactans—found in radishes, tomato, carrot, kiwi, bark of larch
- Are our beautiful plant medicine
- Are not in most animal products
- Inulin—jicama, Jerusalem artichoke; onion & garlic family —leeks, scallions
- Are dietary fibre that acts as a food for the healthy bacteria in your gut. Science has revealed that when there is continually an insufficient amount of prebiotics to feed the probiotics, the gut bacteria will eat the colon itself
- In supplementation form are resilient to stomach HCL, cold, and heat
- May create extensive gas and bloating for people who have SIBO, so what is recommended is working with herbal formulas such as berberine/oil of oregano to rid the small intestine of overgrowth bacteria
- Supplements are often helpful for people with IBS and IBD for when eating fibre is not an option
- Love food that loves us back
- Helpful for metabolic inflammation

## PROBIOTICS:

- Are live bacteria in foods such as sauerkraut and cultured drinks, such as coconut kefir or kvass. When using probiotics, it's essential to research which companies sell viable bacteria—after being shipped and stored. When healing metabolic autoimmune inflammation, not every probiotic will settle well, and a person may need to seek out single-strain probiotics to begin with.

- Bacteria must be kept alive. They may be killed by heat, stomach acid, or simply die with time.

- Are mostly "transient" microbes, as opposed to our "residential" microbes, meaning they come and go. This is why it is necessary to have a daily dose of a probiotic food, (earth food).

- What is news … our resident microbiota is established primarily in first three years.

- In a healthy gut probiotic or commensal bacteria can make up to 85–99% of the gut bacteria, rendering the pathogenic bacteria helpless.

- Compete with the over 1,000 bacteria species already in the gut.

- Love food.

- Helpful for immune regulation. [66,70]

# *Life of Probiotics*

Research has indicated beneficial bacteria along with healing the gut lining reduces inflammation in people with IBD and IBS.

*Lactobacillus plantarum* is one of the main naturally occurring probiotic in sauerkraut and by wildcrafting it with rosehip or wild forage such as juniper berries, we collect more diversity.

"Grace, the soils would plant the antidote - Terrahydrite - for the abuse and rape we do to our soil and plants. It is unbelievable we are surrounded by this level of grace, that nature would have planted 60 million years ago the communication network of a complex microbiome collapse that would survive the last extinction…" Zach Bush, MD

*Culture Me*
*Beyond a germ-phobic reality*
*Back to real sauerkraut, kefirs and brines*
*Kimchi AH, we're free*
*For in brine we trust!*

*Lactobacilli too numerous to count*
*Oh, how much joy you bring me!*
*My microbial mystery*
*Each batch bubbling with unity*

*Colonies to override yeast and disease*
*You set my heart to ease*
*Vitamin Bs of plenty and minerals galore*
*Oh Sauerkraut, Bubbly Sauerkraut!*
*I salt, I score!*
*Producing more and more*
*I soar!*

When you think of making your own sauerkraut, kimchi, fermented (vegan) cheese or yogurt? Do you think it sounds too complicated? And, what does fermented food do for us, anyway?

# Why Ferment & Culture Food?

**FERMENTATION:** Fermentation uses the natural occurrence of salts and bacteria on plants, one known *Lactobacillus plantarum*.

**CULTURE:** Cultured food uses a culture such as kefir grains, yoghurt starter, or a multi-strain pre and probiotic such as a living probiotic.

- Fermentation and culturing is the most ancient way to preserve, store, neutralize unhealthy bacteria, build tons of healthy bacteria, build and assimilate vitamins/minerals and heal digestion through reestablishing what an unhealthy world destroys.

- Microbes were first on earth. They are brilliant beyond belief! They reproduce and give us joy and well-being through the gut/brain connection.

- They reproduce in culture/fermented vegetables, fruit, and through the gut/brain vagus nerve connection—make us feel good.

- The Russian word "kefir" literally means that—to feel good.

- Cultured food is the safest food on our planet. It has been known to quickly heal food poisoning by eating up the bad bacteria. Many people whom have become "fermentistas" have reported an elevation in spiritual consciousness, their connection with Gaia, and REAL food.

When you buy pickles/sauerkraut from a store, most are made from vinegar, not living beneficial bacteria.

Ancient practices encompass chopping, crocks, real highly mineralized salt, and mixing and kneading vegetables to make brine.

## 🫕 Food for Thought:

Almost any veggie can be cultured. Start with the basic sauerkraut and kimchi, then let yourself go wildly into fermentation—forage and add rose hips, juniper berries (I harvest these in the mountains for my kraut), crab apples … and watch your ferment bubble, crunch and pop.

Feel how these ferments satisfy cravings, delight any salad, make great flax crackers, and other side dishes. Added to all meals, cultured vegetables prevent putrefaction of poor food-combining in the gut.

May you all be blessed with a healthy intestinal garden thriving with good microbes.

**Just make sure that all ferments are pressed down tight to release oxygen, that brine covers all vegetable, contents are weighed down, and there is room left in jars for expansion!

In looking at the Human Micorbiome Project (HMP), it is reinforced that beneficial microbes outnumber germ cells 10:1 and that changes in both our lifestyle and the biosphere influence our health and disposition to disease.

The HMP reflects the fact that we are superorganisms composed of human and microbial components, and reflects the notion that rapid, and marked, transformations in human lifestyles are not only affecting the health of the biosphere, but possibly our own health as a result of changes in our microbial ecology.[70]

The HMP has shown that:

- One probiotic cell in the right environment in the gut doubles every 20 minutes. When our microbiota is stressed we have poor nutrition absorption, weight gain, increased risk of diabetes, autoimmune disease, IBD, brain degeneration and cancer. (The key is the right environment).

- The gut epithelial cells have a slower renewal rate in germ-free mice.

- There is a dysregulation in immunity responses, identified in CD and asthma patients, and the link between broad spectrum antibiotics in early childhood and an altered pathogenic microbiome.

- Behaviour differences and neurodevelopmental changes in altered microbial diversity.[70]

## Meditation

Centre yourself and focus on your in-and-out breath. Imagine there is a flourishing garden in your belly. Imagine what would happen when you feed it all nourishment, pure water, and sunshine-mineral-rich living soil. Feel your garden alive, rich, and benefiting you.

Gratitude:

I AM thriving and growing, choosing life.

I AM a microbial-rich, beautiful body electric. As I sink deeply
into this microbial-rich earth, connecting with the microbes of
the grass, trees and air. Blessed, blessed, blessed are we.

I AM....

## Coming Homework

What will you write down as a focused intention for the next seven days?

What pre and probiotic food will you gently add to your life?

What supplementation can you add to your protocol?

What garden can you enrich with living soil?

*Yet only about ten percent of us*
*are nutritionally, metabolically,*
*and biochemically balanced enough*
*to fully benefit from psychotherapy.*
*What's more, years of psychoanalysis*
*or therapy will not reverse the*
*depression that comes from*
*profound omega 3 fatty acids*
*deficiencies, a lack of vitamin B12,*
*a low functioning thyroid,*
*or chronic mercury toxicity.*

**Dr. Gabriel Cousens**[50]

# Chapter 15:

## Supplementation

*Many plant herbal medicines are found on the earth*
*as a gift—dandelion, yarrow, willow …*

### I am not a weed - I am infinite Medicine.

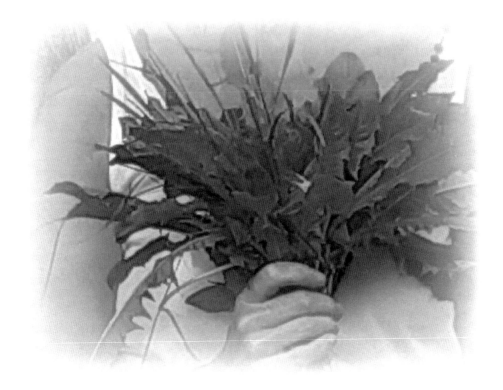

# *Live Food as Medicine & Enzyme Power*

The following supplementation includes examples of what many people with gut issues have used with great success over time. These are suggestions to help you understand that there are many non-invasive healing medicines available to you.

This work is not intended to replace the advice of your medical doctor. Supplementation may no longer be an option. Probiotics are super important! Many functional/integrative doctors have used supplements to assist in healing many things—including depression.

Probiotic foods significantly enrich the enzymatic processes of digestion, as they are predigested foods and assist the microbiome in the assimilation and breakdown of nutrients in medicine food. There are up to a billion actions in our body each second that are dependent on enzymes. Every process requires enzyme activity. Cooked food has lost it enzymes, living food is enzyme-rich–especially if directly from the earth.

Digestive enzymes are protease, lipase and amylase. They may be required less if you are eating live, predigested food, yet are critical when eating cooked food, especially when we understand the putrefaction effect cooked food has on the intestines for people with IBD, yet in acute stages some cooked food is comforting.

Proteolytic / aystemic / metabolic enzymes are the systemic enzymes that eat up the debris—scar tissue, waste, and dead and dying cells. These enzymes alone have been studied as primary healers for many diseases. They allow the body to remove and repair itself in a much more cohesive and effective manner.

Enzyme therapy has been known to have great success rates in healing of many diseases.

Max Wolfe, father of enzyme research, worked with pancreatic enzymes, and had a 95% success rate in healing cardiovascular disease with enzyme therapy.

# Effects of Supplementation on Inflammation

Supplementation may be a catalyst for probiotic synthesis and may no longer be an option. We are bombarded with chemical pollutants everywhere. In order for us to be spiritually inspired, we must feel our body as a thriving organism.

We must have within us the mineral matrix of the earth's ancient life force. In order for us to feel connected to the elements, we require microbial action, enzyme assistance and the synthesis of essential minerals/vitamins found within the elemental matrix of all that is.
Our soil is somewhat depleted on many levels, and many minerals are no longer found in our soil, as well as trace minerals such as: magnesium, iodine, copper, iron, sodium, and boron.

Supplementing minerals is essential to the superconductivity of our body electric. **The root of all disease in traditional medicine is deficiencies and excess**. Deficiencies of any kind can leave us depressed, depleted, anxious, exhausted, and foggy. Some of the most common deficiencies are: B vitamins, selenium, iodine, magnesium, K2, zinc, iron and calcium.

My children ate soil, we all ate food directly out of the garden, my dog is always eating things found in holes in the earth. Effective microorganisms found in the soil feed good bacteria. Most nutrients are absorbed in the intestines and need good bacteria to break them down.

# Mental / Metabolic Supplementation— Anything that Heals the Gut, Heals the Mind

I learned early on, supplementation for healing the intestinal lining:

L-Glutamine, healing herb tea such as licorice and comfrey root as listed below, CBD hemp oil, iodine, GABA, P5P, zinc, taurine, and magnesium. GABA is also required to convert serotonin to N-acetylserotonin. The sleep hormone melatonin is disrupted with in eating conventional food treated with glyphosate. This relaxing feel-good GABA is critical in reducing stress in the gut and stress related issues. For when GABA is low from chronic stress the release of cortisol, nor-epinephrine, and epinephrine elevates glutamate levels, eventually rewiring the body towards stress. GABA is assisted with probiotic bacteria to mediation as most other supplementation is!

When we begin to look at supplementing the microbiome with pre and probiotics, we would be wise to consider warding off the pathogenic bacteria. The microbiome, when being fed, does not distinguish between using fibre to feed pathogenic or commensal bacteria. Individuals suffering from IBD generally have overgrown yeast, fungi and pathogens. In *Listen to Your Gut*, Jini Patel has used a wild oil of oregano protocol as one of her main defences in reestablishing a healthy microbial diversity.[3]

# Herbal Supplementation to Help Rid Imbalanced Pathogenic Bacteria & Heal

All of the following have been very helpful for my healing.

- Wild oil of oregano
- Berberine 200 mg 3x/day
- Garlic
- Caprylic acid
- Grapefruit seed extract
- Structured colloidal silver

## Silver

Colloidal silver has been used for centuries to heal wounds and prevent infections. Its use in healing the bowel is yet unknown. I have used it many times to sooth my digestive tract, settle down a chest infection, and help heal the wounds of my children and animals.

## Hemp CBD oil:

CBD oil can help treat symptoms usually associated with gastrointestinal problems. Some studies even suggest that cannabinoids even help with systemic inflammation that affect our gastrointestinal motility.

## Iodine

Iodine is our greatest detoxifier and pathogenic destroyer. Many people think of iodine as the most important supplement for thyroid health. Often what is less understood, is that iodine is stored in breast tissue, the ovaries and the crypts of the intestines. When we are deficient in iodine, it can be a contributing factor to IBD, ovarian fibroid cysts and other major issues. The importance of iodine supplementation can not be overstressed enough for its abilities to ward off pathogenic bacteria and parasites, help rebuild intestinal lining, healing of the thyroid, decalcification of pineal gland, and aiding us in detoxifying radiation.

## L-butyrate

One of the distinguishable features in people with IBD is that they don't produce enough L-butyrate. L-butyrate supplementation is known to help improve inflammatory markers in people with IBD.

## Vitamin D3

This vitamin has been found to be very helpful in short-term large therapeutic dosage—approximately 5000 IU.

## Aloe Vera

Watch out for preservatives in brands. Using the centre of fresh aloe vera— filleted/ flash-frozen to solidify it—and injected it directly into the colon.

## L-glutamine

Having a fairly large dose of L-glutamine when my intestines feel inflamed, soothed them within a half hour! L-glutamine has been in hospitals as rectal enemas to soothe inflammation. It has a healing and repairing effect on the mucosa lining and works quite quickly for many people.

## Quercetin

## Zinc

Zinc is often one of the deficiencies that people with inflammation or infection have. Zinc helps build the immune system and is critical for cellular repair.

## Deglycerized Licorice (DGL)

## Vitamin A

Every time my blood was tested for minerals and vitamins during acute flare-ups, I was always vitamin A deficient. Vitamin A is predominantly made in the large intestine. Our body's ability to make vitamin A is substantially impaired during chronic inflammation. Vitamin A is paramount for healing and repairing mucosa lining, skin and the overall body. A highly absorbable vitamin A supplement is usually required for many people with IBD.

## B Complex (Especially B12)

Vitamin B complex uses the (complex) combination to work in synergy throughout the body and with other vitamins. Inflammation uses up large amounts of B12. Also, a vegan often requires supplementation of B12. As we become older, it is also common to become deficient in B12, as well. It is wise to use B vitamins on a regular basis and understand their role in mental and gut health. For instance, taking vitamin B3 (niacin) in high doses is known to ward off depression. You may have experienced a refreshing niacin flush when ingesting raw apple cider vinegar.

Hydrochloric acid (HCl) apple cider vinegar in water first thing in the morning prepares the body for digestion.

## Seaweed, spirulina, chlorella, and sprouts,

Support the bioavailability of our biogenetic food. We need sixteen essential and seven trace minerals for life. Your body recognizes algae and sea vegetables as easy protein and minerals.

## Potassium and Electrolytes

Are often depleted in acute intestinal inflammation.

## Prebiotics and Probiotics

In nature and in food are the key that unlocks dormant healing forces. How does the body keep balance, for a functional gut flora is essential for producing, digesting, and assimilating enzymes, allowing nutrients into the body, synthesizing nutrients, such as folic acid, thiamin, and vitamin K (to name but a few), and helping to absorb nutrients, such as calcium, magnesium and iron? BACTERIA!

In her book *The Microbiome Solution,* gastroenterologist Dr. Robynne Chutkan shares the following:

"If you have IBD, optimizing your Vitamin D to a level between 40 and 60 nanograms per millilitre (ng/ml) is an important consideration. Crohn's patients also need to pay attention to vitamin B12, because when your ileum—the end part of your small intestine—is inflamed or has been surgically removed, you cannot absorb B12 as efficiently. Malabsorption of fat-soluble vitamins A, D, E and K, magnesium, iron and more, can also occur. Vitamin D has definitely been shown in many studies to be important for inflammation in general, certainly in patients with IBD. It's one of the first things we check and make sure that people are adequately supplemented." [28]

# Herbs & Gut Health

*Drink your tea slowly, and reverently, as if it is the axis on which the world Earth revolves—slowly, evenly without rushing towards the future. Live the actual moment. Only this moment is life.*

*~ Thich Nhat Hanh*

Medical herbs have been used as long as humans have walked the planet and are establishing themselves in the plant medicine of today. They are respected by indigenous tribes as powerful tonic worthy of our respect and study. The following research is adapted from the author's plant medicine year study with David Crowe.

**GABA** likes carminative herbs such as basil, thyme, peppermint, ginger, cayenne and fermented ginger.

**Ginger**—antiviral. Containing nearly a dozen antiviral compounds, it is also pain-relieving, antiseptic, and antioxidant.

**Echinacea (leaves and flower petals)**—anti-bacterial. Increases levels of properdin, a chemical that activates part of the immune system responsible for increasing defence mechanisms against viral and bacterial attacks.

**Goldenseal**—antiviral, antibacterial, anti-fungal. It is both antiseptic and immune stimulating, increasing blood supply to the spleen. The chemical berberine in goldenseal activates white blood cells that destroy bacteria, fungi, viruses, and tumour cells.

**Sage**—antiseptic, antibacterial. Soothes sore throats, promotes good digestion, and helps ease menstrual cramps.

**Peppermint**—it is not only a painkiller for headaches and reduces fevers by inducing sweating and cooling of the body, but it helps bring up mucus and other material from the lungs, bronchi, and trachea during bronchitis, colds, and the flu.

**Cinnamon**—antibacterial, antiviral, anti-fungal. Helps stop vomiting and relieve nausea, and increases restricted blood flow.

**Clove**—antiviral, anti-fungal, antimicrobial, antioxidant, anti-inflammatory. It helps fight infection and parasites.

**Chamomile**—anti-fungal, antibacterial, antiseptic, anti-inflammatory. Natural sedative.

**Lemongrass**—antibacterial, anti-inflammatory, anti-parasitic, anti-fungal. Relieves digestive ailments and fluid retention, improves blood circulation, and dilates blood vessels.

**Oregano**—a general tonic and immune booster.

**Rosemary**—antibacterial, antiseptic, anti-parasitic, anti-fungal. Good for the nerves and has a stimulating effect.

**Turmeric**—antioxidant, anti-inflammatory, anti-fungal, and anticancer. It is a blood purifier, and helps lower blood sugar levels. Turmeric also turns on BDNF and decreases inflammation.

## Adapted from the Tree of Life Tea for Intestinal Healing Tea

In a pot on the stove, add:

    1 Tbsp slippery elm
    1 Tbsp comfrey root
    1 Tbsp goldenseal
    1 Tbsp marshmallow root
    6 cups water

Bring to a boil. Let steep for 30 – 60 minutes. Strain and drink at room temperature.

## Rameen Yogi Tea

In a large pot, add organic:

  2 Tbsp of fennel seed

  4  cinnamon sticks

  4 Tbsp of dried chaga and/or reishi mushroom

  3 Tbsp of OM tea from Organic Matters

  1 bough of spruce

Fill the pot with water, bring to boil, simmer, and let steep for one hour

# Nature's Supplement: Conscious Eating

So what has happened to us as a society since we have forgotten how to eat for health and what can we do? Alteration in our gut microbes suggests that stress wipes out our happy, sane, peaceful, and loving microbes and innate wisdom, and repair begins the remembering of how to be well and free.

Antibiotics and pesticides are dumped into everything: the food, water, our bodies, the animals we eat. Hundreds of prescriptions are given for every thousand people annually. Chemicals like we have never seen before are circulating everywhere.**What happened?!**

Mouth food, the densest energy source, (air/breath and water being the easily accessible energy forms), if chosen consciously and with right knowledge, can help build spiritual warriors. We need to be spiritual warriors to be resilient in times like these.

How and what we eat has always had a huge impact on body, mind and spirit in a circular continuum. For what we think affects our food choices and our food choices affect how our body feels and how we think—hence, how our spirit interacts with the world. This is true, whether the consumer is conscious of this or not. Food has a causal, biochemical effect. Food is our soon-to-be biology, our quiet friend or foe, our cell building Sattva supply or cell killing choice. Every food choice either sets us free or traps us . What we think, drink, eat has the power to build our bones, blood, brain and breath—circular cause and effect action. Our food choices have the power to be ecologically and compassionately supportive.

Energy follows thought. Stress creates elevated cortisol, adrenalin and inflammatory stress on every system of our cellular matrix. Stress sets us up to emotionally eat. Instead, eat when relaxed!

Even the slightest ingestion of a sensitivity-food can keep our chronic feedback loop of internal inflammation alive. The good news is a live-food, highly mineralized, low-glycemic diet strengthens our immune system and omits the most highly inflammatory and allergenic foods. Our awakened journey, as we study the impact of our food choices, on a multitude of levels, is complex—yet simple. Knowledge is power. Knowing what was programmed around food and drink and choosing to reprogram unhealthy choices can possibly save our lives. Our digestive system is the filtering lenses of every habit, choice and behaviour; both conscious and unconscious.

# Back into the Kitchen & Peace Gardens: The Most Beautiful Supplement of All

*Vegetables, as well as all foods, should be handled and treated with the greatest respect. They are the synthesis of the forces of Heaven and Earth, giving them to us that we can live. They are closer to us than our family and friends, actually transforming themselves into our body and healing us of our sickness. This process is a miracle of miracles and borders on the sacred.*

~ *C. Levin*

Food prepared, with love, quietude, and consciousness, within the natural laws and the practice of gratitude, tastes divine and is healing. Food eaten in a relaxed manner as explained in *Power Eating Program* digests and assimilates easier.

Dr. Gabriel Cousens says he is able to chew each mouthful up to forty times when he connects with the trees, earth, farmers, people, and elements that went into the food—a meditative, peaceful eating practice.

If we live somewhere without space to plant a garden we can sprout sunflowers, mung beans, red clover, fenugreek, and alfalfa—some of my favourites. I teach sprouting in jars, hemp bags, nylon bags and trays. As Steve Meyerowitz shows us in *Sprouts: The Miracle Food*, sprouting is one of the easiest biogenetic foods we can add to our cuisine. It is estimated that sprouts could have 30-1000% more nutrients.

Beautiful pigments of various nutritional value will satisfying taste, balancing live-cultured enzymatic food to create satiation. To this we add the foods that awaken and enrich us. We grow into the addition of healing herbs, conscious growth and prep, and consumption of meals that heal. Knowing our garden, sprouting and using EM and mineral sea agriculture, food co-ops, garden co-ops, community kitchens and food-sharing are all great boosters in our society.

While I write, I have networked—dropping off sauerkraut to some friends today who are too busy to make it. Another friend is growing us sprouts. I am sprouting broccoli sprouts, culturing water, and hitting the farmers market for the next co-op kitchen, drinking EM probiotic, and networking with ancient food as medicine. "I get by with a little help from my friends." This includes my microbial friends as well.

Being prepared is usually the difference between great choices that day, or not such great choices. For myself, always having cultured vegetables and drinks—my dehydrated flax crackers, veggies cut and ready, seeds and nuts sprouted, pates/hummus, and sunflower pate ready to go, is the energy-giver and saver in my life, leading me not into temptation.

As our hormones and biochemistry balance, and our taste buds clear we begin to love bitter, stringent, sour foods—not just salty, fatty, and sweet. The sweets of the past become sickly sweet as we transform.

Eating seasonally and eating the rainbow allows us to get the diversity of nutrients needed. Diversity is the key to our flourishing flora, both in our internal and external gardens.

> *Kill not the food which goes into your mouth. For if you eat living food, the same will quicken you. But if you kill your food, the dead food will kill you also. For life comes only from life, and death comes always from death. For everything which kills your foods, kills your bodies also.*
>
> ~ *The Book of Essenes*

# *FREEDOM FOOD*

*I feed you my beloved*
*"Love food" much different than childhood*
*The raw fats, uncensored and healing—flax, chia, avocado cuisine*
*The pie crusts and pork loins of yesteryear, another lifetime ago it seems*
*Your clean, pure, palate choices refined*
*As you divinely navigate into this moment's perfect platter—a cucumber*
*with some kraut, tomato, avocado, sprouts*
*A bowlful of beauty*

*The inner physician searches for the herbs of heaven—cilantro and parsley*
*today, maybe turmeric tomorrow*

*And we mindfully masticate and contemplate…*
*The farmers, growers, our bellies and bowels*
*Earthly Mother and Father, the sun and the sea*
*And gratefully and humbly*
*Bow and bless her majesty*
*For we are free*
*WE ARE FREE*

# The Happy Gut Summary

How Does Food Affect Our Consciousness? Fast and haphazardous eating is usually reflected in our distracted way of going through life. Eating is part of our meditation practice. Food revolutions have the power to support a society of spiritual beings—on purpose light guides, ecologically awake and compassionate conveyors of the divine.

Why is conscious consumerism essential? In living in deep respect for the planet, each other, and all sentient beings, we create change that heals.

What is conscious living? It is to be aware and fully conscious to what we are doing to the "WHOLE." It means to make feminine-infused, sacred commerce part of the solution in how to maintain consciousness toward Mother Earth. Joseph Campbell would call this "the hero's journey"; Maslow—self-actualization; Dr. Cousens—liberation and living the Six Foundations, Zero-Point, Essenes Sevenfold Peace; Buddha-Nirvana, illumination or empty mind; myself—home, remembering or the miracle mind. We maintain consciousness in all our affairs by continuously evolving and raising up people around us, through joyful living and loving, living by example, sharing amazing nutrient-dense "real happy meals"—not through judgement.

Matt, previous owner of Revolutions in Venice, Los Angeles, said over tea, "There are no 'buts' in conscious commerce, no one is exploited and it is Karma neutral at its very worst, whereas everyday business will sell at the cost of anything—cheaper, faster! And we always pay greater for that!" I believe we feel this deep within our bellies.

Conscious eating is about curiously exploring our diet and developing right dharma, a very intimate lifetime relationship. Food becomes our biology, our prana and changes our biochemistry in such a way we either become energetic, purposeful people, or tired, irritable and acidic—

marked with highs and lows of cellular neurotransmitter depletion.

When daily habits are ones of addictive overstimulation, we are no longer free. We become restless minds, messaging a restless world. remembering if you will.

I have been blessed with three children and now grandchildren. When my children were young I offered them food when they were tired, angry or not well, and they refused the food almost every time. They had better things to do—sleep, express and feel emotions, heal, connect to creation. They were not caught in the pleasure traps yet. They knew how to listen to their bodies long before addictive non-food entered their world. They knew a caterpillar was a far greater fascination than food. It is heartbreaking that this is not the case for most children nowadays. Many are fed addictive food as soon as they begin eating solids, or sooner in utero or breast milk.

Coming home is a continual unravelling of ancestral twine patterning—digesting and sometimes bravely integrating a better way, freeing ourselves to choose from the light. So perhaps conscious eating is an "invitation" to a place beyond disease, addiction, and pharmaceutical surrender as we choose food that accentuates peace: one thought, one prayer, one day at a time.

*This is a food revolution awakening—for the love of our precious Earth, our worth, and the beloved next seven generations unseen.*

## Microbiome Summary

So the question arises, through the lens of the microbiome—both genetic and epigenetic—who is in charge of this inner ecology that lives throughout our digestive tract and satellites all organ systems?

As the microbiome is considered the last organ being studied and recognized now as an essential organ, it is being viewed as the satellite organ involved in all-system physiology, pathology, and health—understanding the individual as the collective and the interface with alterations in health when a microbe population is altered both in our outer and inner gardens.

Again, as in any life altering truth—there is ridicule before truth is accepted as a truth, yet this hypothesis of "the study of one," is quite easy to implement and using "the power of one" to see how quickly one feels better, thinks clearer, and rekindles with childlike joy; as one cultivates love into one's inner garden.

*If we truly understood how essential our microbiome is to regulate every detoxification process, immunity response, neurotransmitter and vitamin synthesis and the control of every inflammatory pathway, we would get "bugged"…with the good stuff.*

This is why the microbiome is also known as our satellite organ. If we remember that everything our gut must assimilate will affect our whole self, everything we eat will either feed us or eat us up, for better or for worse, would we choose "pro life," understanding what we eat, drink, and think as a coevolutionary journey on our way back home?

Would we eliminate the chronic overuse of antibiotics, toxins, stress, toxic-processed food and drink that destroys our beneficial bacteria at alarming rates and is known throughout much research as the greatest negative destroyer of a healthy microbiome?

We are created into this unified field—expressive, diverse and whole. The modern medical model has created many specialists' and separatists' theories that have sometimes created a divided view of how we see ourselves from whole/holy, such as the gut-brain axis of the vagus nerve that affects us bidirectionally, cross-talking with the limbic and endocrine system, primarily from the bottom up.

The incredible neural connection of gut immunity is the receptor field of so much of who we are, connecting us to the heart of the matter. Perhaps our disease-filled world and the imbalance in medical treatment plans are equated to the conduct we have shown Mother Earth—cut it out, poison, expose. This is also known as the Biome Depletion Theory—the wasting of planet Earth is showing up as the wasting of our digestion. Yet there is hope as we remain awake, joining through microbes, searchers of a more compassionate and sustainable way.

Research indicates a healed gut mucosal lining through, whole plant food, highly mineralized, low-glycemic, probiotic diet; stress reduction; natural birth when possible; limited use of antibiotics and EMF exposure, and peaceful loving connection, strengthens our immune system. By omitting the most highly inflammatory foods—sugar, processed foods, allergens, animal products (the highest on the food chain and infused with toxins and pain), gluten, pesticides and chemicals found in all non-organic and genetically engineered food—we can restore our microbiome and begin to reverse dis-ease/metabolic syndromes.

The discovery of the microbiome and the role of bacteria, fungi, and viruses as the body's largest immune regulator, is vast and highly studied in scientific research, with large projects such as the Human Microbiome Project , The Gut Project , Dr. Zach Bush and the M clinic, *The Interconnected Series* with Dr. Pedram Shojai, are changing the way we view every disease today. This new lotus of understanding of the human body from an analysis of homeostasis and health entails consistent practice of "pro life" intake, and the body's ability to suspend, neutralize, and destroy most pathogens, if the microbiome terrain is favourable.

When we finally make a commitment to listen to our gut instincts—feed it a flourishing fauna, frolicking on the grass, ingesting microbial truths—while freeing our children from nature deprivation and a processed life, we may have discovered the "fast track" to holistic wellness, brain restoration and a connection so old and deep that separation disappears into the microbial web of dynamic mystery.

## Give Gratitude Light not Heat: An Ending Blessing

"I get by with a little help from my friends" —both microbial and human/animal ones, then sometimes a gentle reminder on the next breeze comes, and "we are not just dust in the wind but rather recycled light, stardust, and transmuting energy." Meditation helps us ground our love into a world so in need of this. Maybe we just are simply recycled stars as pondered in a prose poem my friend John shared:

*The stars were formed*
*roughly at first*
*In giving of their light*
*Once finished*
*Can fragment*

*We are not perfect*
*And some souls leave early*
*Yet, we can still give light through love*
*Restoring ourselves in thankfulness*
*For simple things…*

Let us marvel in thankfulness. Matter and light are interchangeable. My wise friend John once said, *"Marvel my child at how photosynthesis creates life from light."*

Photosynthesis is the process in which plants, some bacteria and some protistans use the energy from sunlight to produce glucose from carbon dioxide and water, converted into pyruvate, release adenosine triphosphate (ATP) via cellular respiration. Hence, oxygen is formed. Light is infinite and spacious attractor energy, a lighthouse if you will. Light respects sovereignty, a state in which we recognize we have autonomy over ourselves, and the power and responsibility to rule all aspects of our lives; creating flow and a safe harbour. Rameen Peyrow tells us, our job here is to keep our mindbody temple pure so our soul may shine through brightly!

What exactly is giving light, not heat? It is a world of non-codependency, right action and non-conflict. For its opposites attract heat, heat as inflammatory thoughts and a belly on fire. This light, when ignited, burns up the rubbish. It is the kind of fire in the belly that ignites the Tan Tien, and shines so bright that it allows others to find their way, beginning the thousand-mile journey home towards remembrance.

In the beautiful literary art of Lars Muhl in The *Gate of Light*, he describes an ancient healing method used by the Essenes, or The Sons of Light, 2500 years ago, as the living prayer of our hearts and an open hand offering of heart-light to another.

Yes, that bright lighthouse scans across the seas, letting its presence be known. Illumination may be the key to our survival, putting out the driving force of all inflammation, keeping our face to the sun, until darkness no longer can do anything other than reveal shadow. Surrendering to the present moment, one healing change at a time, is the spice of life.

We are in a health crisis on this planet. It is more essential than ever to protect our health and to awaken. We free up so much energy to live in health when our connection is rooted in connecting back to our land. We can no longer believe politicians or food safety regulatory bodies. We are the ones who will make the change. If nothing changes, nothing changes!

As we turn our brains back on, we have the opportunity to look around and say, "Hey, what the bleep is happening?" Gandhi had made a commitment to make one dietary change every four months. What will you change? How would our lives change if we chose to release one proinflammatory choice each month and add in an anti-inflammatory, alkalizing choice in its place? Imagine starting our morning with meditation, green juice, turmeric tea, combining comfrey, slippery elm and horsetail to soothe the colon.

Lino Stanchich sums this up nicely in *Power Eating Program*: "Eating is the act of creating your body, your very life. What more important act do we perform daily? What more profound way do we honor and love ourselves?"

Our awakened journey is complex yet simple. Knowledge is power. Knowing what was programmed around food, drink and our nutrition and choosing to reprogram unhealthy choices, may save our precious EarthGut. When we are at peace with our bodies we have found a diet that promotes "ahimsa"—peace of mind and non-harm. We choose infused cuisine, rich in both plant fibre and microbial builders. More and more community gardens are being built, organic food is found everywhere and information is being shared. This is a great change! This is awakened Love.

Individualizing our diet, along with practising our own style of meditation enables us to connect intuitively with our individual nutritional requirements. This gets deeper and deeper over time and may be the most conscious, creative way into a deep level of self-trust and empowerment. In this space; every meal is a blessing, every moment an opportunity. This deepening connection can't help but overflow to all other areas of our lives.

By filling our bodies with food from the "light menu," we confidently navigate away from the pull of less-than-optimal food, lifestyle distractions, and acidic drinks. We are able to deeply listen to that quiet voice that directs us to the unique healing foods, for our specific biochemistry. Over time our intuitive "knowing" of the correct food for our medicine, comes more and more naturally. Our cells die, regenerate or rearrange with every breath, therefore so does the energy and nutrition needs.

*We are light returning to light.*
*Most valuable, is experiencing our every breath*
*as a reminder we do belong here at*
*this time—to love and be loved.*

*May we clear away all that no longer shines,*
*exhale it, and breathe life into the shadows*
*of our beautiful souls—separation and lack illusions,*
*evaporating back into nothingness!*

*May we all be blessed with the beauty way*
*of giving light and not heat.*

*May we all have the strength and self-love to explore*
*inflammation and it's root causes.*

*May all sentient beings be happy and free!*

# Juice & Liquid Recipes

## Dietary Suggestions for Liquid Bowel Rest: Conscious Eating & Mindful Mastication

*In the market I walk*
*Through the garden I enter*
*Reverence it asks …listen*

*To the food I ask*
*To the seeds my saliva ignites*
*To the tables I bring thee*
*Laughter, renewal, connection*

*Let us always listen*
*To what the food is offering*
*Let us bring forth to the people*
*Food as medicine, food as love*

## Ahimsa & Hope: Food as Love, Peace and Inspiration

Conscious eating gets deeper and deeper over time and may be one of the most conscious, creative ways into a deeper level of self-trust, self-confidence, and feeling truly empowered. In this space, every meal is a blessing, every food an opportunity. This deepened connection and loving lifestyle can't help but overflow to all other areas of your life.

Filling our refrigerators and bodies with food we feel amazed about allows us to make peace within ourselves, and less-than-optimal food and drink no longer has a hold on us. We are able to deeply listen to that quiet voice that directs us to the unique healing foods for our biochemistry, in that very moment. Over time, this becomes more and more natural. It is our birthright to be happy, healthy, and free.

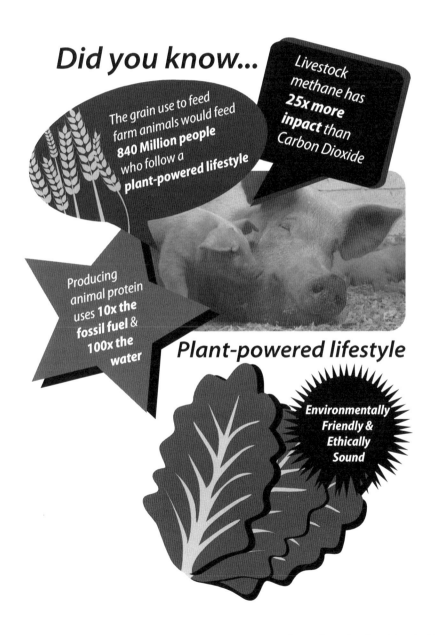

# CRAVING SUBSTITUTES

| If you crave this… | | These healthy foods contain it: |
|---|---|---|
| **Chocolate** | | Raw nuts and seeds, legumes, fruits |
| **Sweets** | | Broccoli, grapes, dried beans |
| | | Fresh fruits |
| | | Nuts, legumes, grains |
| | | Cranberries, horseradish, cruciferous vegetables, kale, cabbage |
| | | Raisins, sweet potato, spinach |
| **Bread, toast** | | High protein foods such as nuts, beans |
| **Oily snacks, fatty foods** | | Mustard and turnip greens, broccoli, kale, legumes, sesame |
| **Coffee or tea** | | Nuts, legumes |
| | | Red peppers, garlic, onion, cruciferous vegetables |
| | | Himalayan salt, apple cider vinegar (on salad) |
| | | Seaweed, Atlantic dulse, greens, black cherries |
| **Alcohol, recreational drugs** | | Nuts |
| | | Mustard and turnip greens, broccoli, kale, legumes, vegan cheese, sesame |
| | | Supplement glutamine powder for withdrawal, raw cabbage juice |
| | | Sun-dried black olives, potato peel broth, seaweed, bitter greens |

| | | |
|---|---|---|
| **Chewing ice** | | Seaweed, greens, black cherries |
| **Burned food** | | Fresh fruits |
| **Soda and other carbonated drinks** | | Mustard and turnip greens, broccoli, kale, legumes, sesame |
| **Salty foods** | | Himalayan salt, raw flax crackers |
| **Acid foods** | | Raw nuts and seeds, legumes, fruits |
| **Preference for liquids rather than solids** | | Flavour water with lemon, lime or raw apple cider vinegar. Remember: 8 to 10 glasses per day |
| **Preference for solids rather than liquids** | | You have been so dehydrated for so long that you have lost your thirst. Flavour water with lemon, lime or raw apple cider vinegar. Remember: 8 to 10 glasses per day |
| **Cool drinks** | | Walnuts, almonds, pecans, pineapple, blueberries |
| **Premenstrual cravings** | | Leafy vegetables, root vegetables |
| **General overeating** | | Nuts, seeds; avoid refined starches |
| | | Raisins, sweet potato, spinach |
| | | Vitamin C supplements or orange, green, red fruits and vegetables |
| **Lack of appetite** | | Nuts, seeds, beans |
| | | Seeds and legumes |
| | | Walnuts, almonds, pecans, pineapple, blueberries |
| | | Himalayan salt |

# Getting in the Gap: Chew, CHEW

Sometimes there's a gap between what we know and what we do… Hmmm… have you ever experienced this, I know I have! :) It's helpful to find the humour and be gentle with ourselves on this journey to the "light menu."

Jungian therapists may call this our shadow, Kabbalistic Jewish may call this the opponent/ backlash or Buddhists may call this the hungry ghosts, yet, one thing is for certain—when we bring breathful mindfulness to mindless eating and consuming, we have an opportunity to interrupt and upgrade our destructive patterns.

The deep full mindbody connection to food that we have acquired since birth is one of incredible intimacies. When we fully commit to upgrading our nutrition we may come face to face with much opposition, both externally and internally.

Being peaceful and gentle with ourselves during this transition, allowing the "fast-track" and allowing the incredible recipes and foods to become the "proof in the chia pudding." When our bodies began to upgrade from the "light menu" we feel more alive and whole. The shift towards plant-based nutrition is growing astronomically fast for both health and planetary concerns.

*With the angels of infinite love and gratitude, I commit to mindfully masticate every magical mouthful of my blessed living cuisine—33 times.*

Much research has been done on the power of chewing our food thoroughly. Research has shown us that mindful mastication creates relaxation responses, and allows us to connect and feel blessed with all the energy and care that has gone into our food. There has been research on how chewing our food slowly and thoroughly has even allowed some people to live and survive in concentration camps, extracting the most nutrition out of their food as possible. When we make eating a meditation practice, we may access divine digestion by connecting with the trees, the gardens and the people involved with our food. Thoroughly chewing our food also allows us to be more connected to when we have had enough to eat and to only eating until we are 70% full.

Eating consciously means we eat for peace and protection for all—first and foremost. It means live-food clears us, so we may do our work, the work of AWAKENING. By eating consciously we become more intuitive and can tap into our ever-changing body electric and modify, shift, and fine-tune our eating, each and every moment. Can we all jump right in and never look back, always choosing from the "light" menu? As many teachers tell us, we need to just keep turning ourself back into the right direction.

We learn through observation. As children we are in theta, the hypnotic state until approximately seven years of age. We learn through watching. Therefore, we must be gentle with ourselves as we reprogram. We must use the power of grace and stay connected with like-minded souls who are way showers of liberation.

# Gratitude Heals

Enjoy every bite. Saying yum (or your version of this) and thank you while you eat and drink will increase the healing properties of our nutritious food. The book *Messages From Water* helps us understand the importance of sending positive messages to our water body electric.

Love and gratitude are first on the list of ingredients, as they are the most important. Love and gratitude are the most transformational ingredients on the planet! When we breathe in love and gratitude, we impact our central nervous system and shift our brain chemistry to a more happiness-friendly environment. When we add love and gratitude to our experience around our relationship with food, it is profoundly transformational!

# Benefits of Live, Raw, Organic, Veganic, Non-GMO Food

## 🍲 Food for Thought:Enzymes are Life!

Live/raw food is used interchangeably in this work. The phrase "living food" means enzymes and nutrition are not destroyed in the uncensored form.

There are thousands of food enzymes and phytonutrients out there, but we are only knowledgeable of about 2,000 of them. However, there is one thing for certain, heat changes them all and cooking depletes the nutrients from the food and contributes to human illness.

Now I know, as with any good argument, there are two sides. There have been claims that raw food causes digestive issues and bloating. If this is an issue you face, you can try increasing the number of times that you chew your food. The optimal amount of "chews" has been listed between 50 and 80, depending on the food you're eating. Think about it like this ... the more digestion done in our mouth, the easier it will be for the digestion in our stomach!

Not only is there a depletion in the nutrient content, but the exposure to high temperatures actually increases carcinogens, which is dangerous to human health, because this process destroys so much of the nutrient content, our bodies trigger greater appetite to get more food in order to get the necessary nutrients. This naturally leads to diseases like obesity and diabetes since the foods consumed are essentially empty calories.

If cooking in oil, the oil itself actually loses its antioxidant properties. The structure of fat cells is shifted from cis to trans. In other words, the actual fat molecules in our food are going from good to bad. When food is cooked, so many changes begin happening, and not in a good way.

*Although there is some debate when it comes to digestion, overall you will get more nutrients and greater health benefits from food in its most natural, raw state."*

***The Tree of Life Rejuvenation Center***

Along with limiting the amount of cooked food that is consumed,. we also remove:

Refined sugar: Causes insulin resistance and fatty liver. Strong links to obesity, diabetes and heart disease.

Refined grains: Lead to rapid spikes in blood sugar, insulin resistance and weight gain. Strong links to many chronic, Western diseases.

**Vegetable oils:** High in inflammatory Omega-6 fatty acids, increase inflammation and oxidative damage.

**Trans fats:** Extremely harmful, man-made fats found in processed foods and linked to many serious diseases, especially heart disease

**Processed foods:** Low in nutrients and high in harmful ingredients.

## 🐢 Food for Thought: Why Organic & Veganic

Veganic farms use only plant-based fertilizers, together with smart growing techniques such as alternating crops over time to build nutrients in the soil. Veganic is a step beyond organic, a step toward greater purity, greater health benefits and a safer food supply. Organic farming may still use animal waste fertilizer, which may still have contaminants found in animal products.

- More beneficial nutrients
- Fresher: not sprayed with preservatives and aren't stored for months at a time.
- Less allergy-stimulating, fewer chemicals to irritate sensitive systems.
- Fewer pesticides. The chemicals in non-organic foods, such poisons as: fungicides, herbicides, and insecticides, are not just on the peel of the food, the plants actually pull these chemicals through their vascular systems.
- Grown in soil with its natural flora and nutrients intact.
- More environmentally sound: Organic farming practices reduce pollution, conserve water, reduce soil erosion, increase soil fertility, and use less energy. Farming without pesticides is also better for nearby birds and animals as well as people who live close to the farms.
- GMO-free WATER purified, non-chlorinated water, remineralized, non-fluorinated

| Heavily Sprayed Foods | Less Sprayed Foods |
|---|---|
| Apples | Asparagus |
| Celery | Avocado |
| Cherry Tomatoes | Cabbage |
| Cucumbers | Cantaloupe |
| Grapes | Corn (GMO-Free) |
| Hot Peppers | Eggplant |
| Nectarines | Grapefruit |
| Peaches | Kiwi |
| Potatoes | Mangos |
| Spinach | Mushrooms |
| Strawberries | Onions |
| Sweet Bell Peppers | Papaya |
| Kale | Pineapple |
| Collard Greens | Sweet Peas |
| Summer squash (including Zucchini) | Sweet Potato (GMO-Free) |
| Coffee Beans | |
| Tea Leaves | |
| Almonds | |

# *Food Combining*

Follow the food-combining guidelines in order to maximize your detoxification and digestion.

## Only Combine Circles that Touch

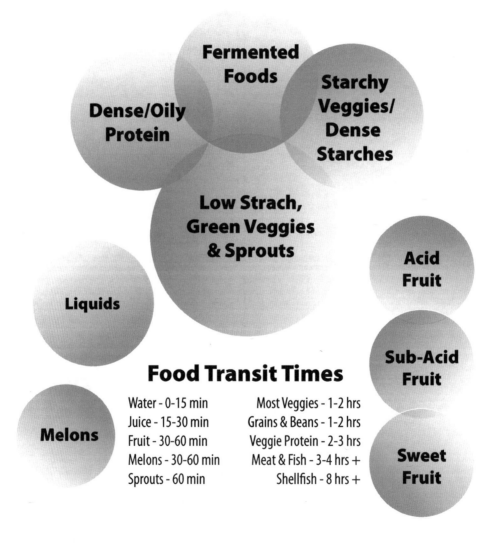

Fermented Foods

Dense/Oily Protein

Starchy Veggies/ Dense Starches

Low Strach, Green Veggies & Sprouts

Acid Fruit

Liquids

Sub-Acid Fruit

### Food Transit Times

| | |
|---|---|
| Water - 0-15 min | Most Veggies - 1-2 hrs |
| Juice - 15-30 min | Grains & Beans - 1-2 hrs |
| Fruit - 30-60 min | Veggie Protein - 2-3 hrs |
| Melons - 30-60 min | Meat & Fish - 3-4 hrs + |
| Sprouts - 60 min | Shellfish - 8 hrs + |

Melons

Sweet Fruit

Each food type requires digestion enzymes and length of time to digested. Combining foods that are complimentary aids assimilation of nutrients as well as avoids putrefaction of food in the intestines.

## Note:

- Only combine low-glycemic vegetables with fruit.
- Always eat melons separate.
- Never mix fruit with oily, starch and protein foods; i.e.,
  Nuts, seeds and avocados.
- Eat citrus fruits separately.
- Drink water 5-10 minutes before meals and 1-2 hours after meals.
- Sweet fruits such as bananas and apples in your smoothie should only be mixed with low-starch vegetables such as lettuce, cucumber, celery.
- The key to making any healthy choice, is to be prepared and to set yourself up for success!
- Always having a wide selection of choices to not only keep fuel in the tank, but that actually fit your specific cravings. This will go a long way towards creating the new eating habits that you are wanting to put into place.
- Think about what you crave. When you get hungry, when is it most likely that you will reach for a food that you would rather replace?
- Children love veggies and dips!
- Always have a selection of veggies and vegan living dips available!

# Centring in Love and Gratitude:

Take a moment now and breathe in love and gratitude. Breathe in love and gratitude for your willingness to investigate new choices and a lifestyle that will bring you health, greater energy and the peace that you truly crave. Breathe in love and gratitude and allow it to create space inside of your being. Breathe in love and gratitude and allow it to expand that tight container that you have been living in. Breathe in love and gratitude and feel your body's desire for vibrant nutrition, for loving care and for deep connection. Breathe in love and gratitude and experience what it's like to feel present with your breath. Breathe in love and gratitude and feel the clarity and ease of being here and now. Breathe in love and gratitude and welcome this moment for exactly what it is.

# The "Fast" Track

*Fasting is the first principle of medicine.*

*Rumi*

## What's Really Happening Here? Moving Beyond the Deprivation Mindset. Let's Think about This:

In our bodies we have all our systems sending messages to us, telling us what is needed and the status of their functionality, through feelings of hot, cold, tingling, pain, pleasure, our mood, hunger … even things like the urge to pee is a status report from our body. We get countless signals every day and we are constantly adjusting ourselves to accommodate this feedback. Imagine yourself at a very noisy event, with lights flashing, people moving around you, hundreds of people talking, music playing, kitchen noises, the smell of the people and food; there's no way that you hear, see, smell, feel, taste everything all at once. Most of us have the ability to block out a great deal of the noise to be able to focus (mostly) on what is in front of us, what we've decided as important. It's the same within our bodies, except we've gotten too good at blocking out the signals our bodies have been giving us. We are missing essential messages. Fasting has the ability to clear out all of the overstimulation in our digestive tract. Cleansing allows us to reset our telomeres, fears and intuition. Telomeres are the caps on our chromosomes, which become depleted as we age.

Scientific bodies of work have connected calorie restriction, intermittent fasting, and fasting as some of the quickest ways to activate our anti-aging genes.

What is a green juice fast? It is drinking only green juice without sugar, such as the recipes below, fasting juice vs. cleansing juice. Cucumber, celery, sprout juice will allow the body to stay in a fasting mode while cleansing, upping the epigenetic blueprint and allowing the body to go into auto-ketosis, which means that the body is able to burn fat instead of glucose. In this state the body is able to get rid of debris and burn up the rubbish.

## *Even a 24 hour fast will:*

- Activate a multitude of anti-aging genes
- Begin to clean out the colon
- Begin to break overeating/addictive food patterns
- The research of "indican bowel toxicity" testing tells us that a seven day green juice fast rids the bowel of most if not all toxins.

## *Points to Ponder Regarding Fasting:*

- Honouring the "law of readiness" when it comes to fasting:
- For most people, setting themselves up for success when fasting usually looks like unplugging from "busy-ness" and carving out 3–7 days just to juice, rest, and reset. For many people, eliminating solid food is challenging and people find having support very beneficial when they begin fasting. This may be done with a partner, a nutritional counsellor, a rejuvenation centre, and/or connection to a higher divine source through quietude, rest, and readiness.
- Being prepared is extremely important.

- Purchasing all food and supplies for juicing ahead of time, having a ready supply of green juice, herbal teas and purified water to nourish yourself with. Also ensuring you have other fasting supporters: enema bag (colon cleansing is very important during a fast) and even a journal to write in.
- A seven-day green juice fast will keep your blood sugar balanced, reset your telomeres, remove bowel toxicity, and upgrade your body chemistry, this results in non-causal happiness (happiness for no reason, unreasonable happiness)
- Many health practitioners, have used fasting as a way to heal themselves and their clients. For instance: Dr. Bernard Jensen healed his prostate cancer through fasting. Anne Wigmore healed her IBD and other systemic illnesses through green juice fasting and the use of wheatgrass, thereby founding the use of wheatgrass as it is used across the globe today.
- The Essenes use seven-day fasting to release negativity.
- Fasting has had the ability to help heal the root cause of all misaligned eating.
- We can customize juicing to fit our lives. When we realize that everything matters, we realize that intermittent fasting, one day of fasting, three to seven days of fasting … and beyond has the ability to significantly upgrade our health towards living a dis-ease free life.
- Intermittent fasting means shortening the time per day that we are putting calories into the body.
- Consider Fasting for The Seasons: Spring and Fall are the body's most receptive times to clean house.
- Earth often lends her medicinal herbs at this time, the ones that are most restorative to flush liver, bowel and whole-body toxins, are the large amount of dandelion greens given to us so generously in the spring. I invite you to connect with the weeds of spring and fall,

to allow yourself to connect with their medicine. When we clear the toxins from our bodies, we have a deeper connection with what the earth so generously donates. This connection may look like a release from annihilating all that's good in our systems, to releasing our need to use poison, such as chemical weed killers, that have a horrific effect on the oneness of our planet.

- When people have seasonal allergies, they often get the most relief from doing a cleanse. Cleansing allows us to discover the direct correlation to releasing ingested toxins/allergens, to the body's ability to not overreact to external allergens. It is often in the spring and fall that we want to cleanse the cobwebs and excess stuff in our homes. If we overlook the home that is our body, we are missing out on the most significant piece of cleansing.

## Fasting Options:
## Intermittent Fasting:

Is a great way to upgrade our entire mindbody. Shortening the window of time each day in which we ingest calories. This allows the digestive system and whole body to rest, detoxify and reset within every 24 hour period. It's often practised between 14–18 hours per day

For example: 6:00 p.m. – 12:00 p.m. the next day of calorie restriction, green juice, herbal tea, water fasting then eating light meals between 12 p.m. and 6 p.m.

## Customized Juice Fasting for Your Life

Remember: Everything matters—every piece of the puzzle matters!

To echo what we started this book with, each cleansing choice adds up. So, choosing to do any juicing will add nutrients, detoxify and is another step in a healthy direction. Let's celebrate each step.

From one juice a day, to juice cleansing for one, three, five, seven, or even twenty-one days, you can work with your body, nutritional counsellor and medical professional to choose what is right for you.

This is where listening and turning up the volume on the subtle messages your body is giving you will pay off. The more you juice cleanse, the more attuned to your body's messages you will be. Your body knows best; there is a very different experience between the yeast in your body crying out for sugar and your body's wisdom telling you that you have had enough time inside of your fast. Go at your own pace and while it's important to have goals, fasting isn't a process of having enough "willpower"; it's a process of listening to, loving, and becoming reacquainted with your body's natural rhythm and real nutritional needs. Every single person that I have witnessed in healing centres and as a practitioner, has seen incredible changes in both the physical, mental, and emotional bodies with fasting!

# Liquid Love:
## Juice, Smoothies,
### Healing Tea & Elixirs

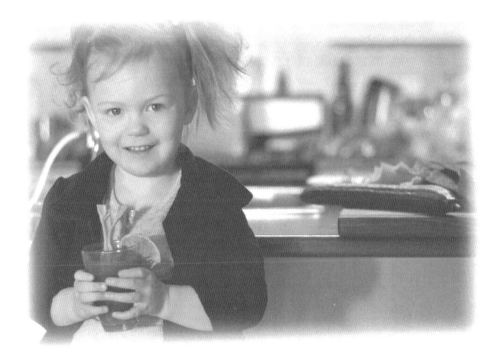

Food for thought: If you have a job in which you hurry, consider bringing a lunch that mainly consists of liquid love recipes. All recipes are made with FRESH, RAW, ORGANIC ingredients. YUM!

# JUICE

*Remember: If your limes and lemons are organic, juice the rind along with the fruit*

## CELERY only JUICE
*as recommended by Anthony Williams in The Medical Medium*

> Juice 2 celery bunches
>
> Makes approximately 2 cups of juice
>
> Drink first thing in the am for gut healing

## BASIC GREEN
*Daily supply for someone who is juicing*

> 5 cucumbers
>
> 1 head celery
>
> 1 lemon or lime
>
> Optional: 1 green apple

## GREEN JUICE for INTERMITTENT FASTING
*Daily supply for someone who is juicing*

> 5 cucumbers
>
> 1 head celery
>
> ½ lemon or lime
>
> Can dilute with water

## APPLE OF MY EYE

½ apple
3–4 stalks of celery
1 cucumber
½ tsp apple cider vinegar
Optional: 1 tsp greens powder

## FRESH GREEN

1 apple
1 cucumber
½ bunch of cilantro
sprig of fresh basil

## GREEN DRINK

*Preferably in the afternoon, drink 10 ounces freshly juiced green vegetables: cucumber, parsley, spinach, kale, celery, or any other green herb or vegetable.*

Add fresh lemon juice and/or freshly juiced ginger to pep up the flavour. Fresh mint also makes a nice addition with cucumber and other milder-tasting greens.

## THE REVITALIZER

2 tomatoes
½ lemon or lime, peeled
½ cucumber, peeled
6 to 8 string beans

*Cut produce to fit juicer feed tube. Juice ingredients and stir. Pour into a glass and drink as soon as possible.*

## MOOD MENDER

3 fennel stalks, including leaves and flowers

2 stalks celery

½ pear

3 carrots, scrubbed well, tops removed,

½ - inch chunk ginger, scrubbed, ends trimmed or peeled if old

*Cut produce to fit juicer feed tube. Juice ingredients and stir.*
*Pour into a glass and drink as soon as possible.*
*Note: Fennel juice has been used as a traditional tonic to help the*
*body release endorphins, the "feel good" peptides, from the brain into*
*the bloodstream. Endorphins help to diminish anxiety, fear*
*and generate euphoria.*

## PEPPY PARSLEY

1 bunch parsley

½ cucumber, peeled

2 celery stalks

½ lemon, peeled

1 to 2 carrots, scrubbed well, tops removed, ends trimmed

## GRATITUDE GINGER

5 cucumbers

1 head celery

1 lemon or lime

1 green apple

1 inch ginger

## *VEGETABLE JUICE RATIOS*

### REGULAR JUICE PROPORTIONS PER 12 oz

5 oz Cucumber

2 oz Zucchini

3 oz Celery

1 oz Cabbage

1 oz Carrot

Sprouts

### LOW-GLYCEMIC JUICE PROPORTIONS PER 12 oz

6 oz Cucumber

2 oz Zucchini

3 oz Celery

1 oz Cabbage

Sprouts

# SMOOTHIES

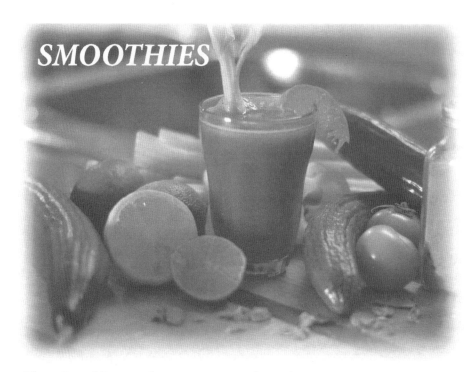

*Plant-Based Protein Suggestions - Brad King's Protein & SunWarrior, Hemp Infinity 8 protein: Listen to your body as to what resonates!*

Blueberries: can be exchanged with any low-glycemic berry such as raspberry, blackberry, sour cherry, and cranberry

## ELECTROLYTE HIGH CALORIE FOR IBD HYDRATION

1 litre of organic fresh juice of celery
blend with 2 bananas

## MY FAVOURITE HYDRATION DRINK

Juice 4 celery slacks
one whole organic lemon and lime
in one litre of water ½ tsp. himalayan salt

## BASIC BLUEBERRY

½ cup frozen blueberries (or other low-glycemic berry)

1 cup celery & cucumber juice

1 Tbsp hemp protein powder

1 Tbsp ground flax

*Optional: small handful of mixed greens*

*1 tsp greens powder*

## SMOOTHIE FOR TWO

1 cup frozen blueberries

1 cup cucumber pulp

1 scoop plant-based protein powder

¼ – ⅓ cups hemp hearts

3 – 4 cups water

*Optional: Sweeten to taste with low-glycemic sweetener such*
*as lakanto or stevia*

## NUTTY RASPBERRY SMOOTHIE

½ cup frozen raspberries

½ cup cucumber pulp

1 scoop plant-based protein powder

⅓ cup sprouted almonds

2 cups water

*Optional: 1 tsp almond butter*

*Sweeten to taste with low-glycemic sweetener such as lakanto or stevia*

## PULPERY BLUEBERRY BLISS SMOOTHIE

½ cup frozen blueberries

½ cup cucumber pulp

1 scoop plant-based protein powder

1 cup cashew-sesame mylk

½ cup cashew-sesame mylk pulp

2 cups water

*Optional: Sweeten to taste with low-glycemic sweetener such*
*as lakanto or stevia*


## GREEN MINT SMOOTHIE

1½ cup almond mylk

1½ cup water

12 organic mint leaves

1½ cup spinach or kale or a 50/50 mix

2 Tbsp organic raw almond butter or almond pulp

1 Tbsp or more organic raw coconut nectar

*For extra low-glycemic replace the coconut nectar with 5 drops of stevia.*

# Blend it up and enjoy!

Drinking medicinal herbs, green juices and blended food is a beautiful and nourishing way to easily assimilate and connect to ourselves, the divine and others. Tea rituals have been performed and continue to be mindfully practised around the world.

Many people are discovering the art and joy in liquid elixirs, the sipping of a high-quality herbal tea, sweet fresh almond mylk made fresh or a nutritional smoothie. Smoothies have become a common food for many people on the go. Yet, many are full of sugars, highly processed protein powders and combinations that are sure to imbalance blood sugar and energy levels. May we explore a new way to look at liquid love food, that will love you back, that is both satisfying and balancing.

## Discover:

1.  Mixing and matching herbs to any drink
2.  Adding good healthy fat to a smoothie enriches the flavour, enhances energy, keeps the body balanced and creates satisfaction. Such as adding avocado, raw almond butter, nuts, seeds and coconut oil
3.  Adding high protein food will provide you sustained energy over the day. Such as spirulina, chlorella, nuts, seeds, spinach and other delicious greens
4.  Sipping a warm beverage such as an elixir, miso broth or peppermint tea can support digestion and add warmth to a raw meal during the cold months.
5.  A glass of fresh green juice is energizing, satisfying and detoxifying, all in one!

May we all be joyful in our endeavours, knowing liquid food is an amazing way to access nutrition in all situations, and considerably more so when time for mindful mastication is not available.

If experiencing extreme gut inflammation, a Claymonde fast is recommended for 1–3 days. This recipe has kept many people out of the hospital despite terrible diarrhea and vomiting. The elements in this recipe soak up the toxins in the gut, keep up the electrolytes and act as a prebiotic, encouraging the growth of the good bacteria. Use only glass cups or jars and wooden spoons, as the clay may pick up undesirable ions from plastic and metal.

## CLAYMONADE

¾ litre of filtered water

1 heaping Tbsp of French green clay

1 heaping Tbsp of raw honey

2 lemons, squeezed

Good quality honey is hard like a rock. If you can pour your honey, it is heated and the enzymes destroyed and it is useless to help you. Dissolve the honey with the water, or transfer to a blender and blend it (I sometimes pour a cup of filtered water into my honey pail overnight to dissolve it), put water and honey into a glass jar, add the clay and squeezed lemon juice, stir with a wooden spoon, and drink as needed. This is often a great way to start the day as the body goes through a cleansing cycle in the mornings.

# ELIXIRS

There is no limit to what you can do with elixirs, these are soothing and nutritionally power packed beverages!

## Basic Elixir Instructions

Put dry ingredients into Vitamix first, then add water and strain all elixirs through mylk bag, easy peasy.

General Nut and Seed Mylk suggestions

Blend:

1 cup overnight soaked nuts or seeds to 3 cups water

Options:

Almond extract

Vanilla extract

Cinnamon extract

½ tsp natural sweetener

## ALMOND MYLK

1 cup sprouted almonds (soaked 12 to 24 hours and rinsed)

Blend with 3 cups of water

Pour into pulp bag, milk bag (as if milking a cow) into another container

Add vanilla to taste

Add a pinch of Himalayan salt

*Optional: Yacon syrup or stevia to sweeten the taste*

## CASHEW-SESAME MYLK

1 cup cashews

1 cup sesame

4 cups water

*Optional: 2 tbsp yacon syrup (to sweeten the taste)*

## COCONUT MYLK

1 cup shredded coconut

3½ cup water

Blend at high speed for 1 minute

## LIQUID GOLD

3 cups nut, seed or coconut mylk

3 tsp turmeric

*Optional: natural sweetener to taste*

## COCO CHAGA LOVE

3 cups richly steeped chaga

1 cup nut or seed mylk

1- 2 tbsp carob powder

1 tbsp natural sweetener

*Optional:*

*1 tsp cinnamon*

*1 tsp Cardamom*

*For diabetics we suggest replacing cocoa with carob, as cacao has been found to increase blood sugar

### 🍵 Food for Thought:

Chaga has been known to Native people as a powerful medicine for a long time. Chaga grows on birch trees in northern climates and is known as one of the most medicinal, anti-disease, adaptogen, a food that helps us adapt to stress, both environmental and emotional in origin. In the past, reishi mushroom has been given a lot of press, now we understand that chaga is even a more powerful plant-food medicine. The black-rich colour of the chaga adds to our "jing" or life force.

## GUT HEALER

1 tsp Slippery Elm

1 tsp Comfrey Root

1 tsp Marshmallow root

1 tsp Licorice root

6 cups water

Bring to Boil

Let steep for 30 min – 1 hour

Strain and drink at room temperature

## MOUNTAIN MINT ELIXIR

1 cup peppermint tea

1 cup nut or seed milk

4-5 fresh mint leaves

4-5 drops mint extract

*Optional: Use natural sweetener to taste*

Blend and top with a mint leaf

To serve cool, add ice before blending

## SOLEIL SAGE-MINT TEA

½ cup sage leaves

10 mint leaves

1 peppermint/ spearmint tea bag

*Optional: Use natural sweetener to taste*

Fill 2 L jar with water, sage, mint and tea ingredients.

Cover jar and place in sunlight for full day

Strain

Add sweetener

This also may be done with hot water. Serve chilled or hot

Make into an elixir by blending 1 up of this tea with 1 cup of nut or seed mylk and sweetener of choice

## *GINGER LEMONADE*

2 inch piece of ginger

2 lemons

1½ litre of water

*Optional: Natural sweetener to taste*

Juice ginger with lemons, including the rinds (of organic lemons)

Serve chilled

*If you would like to make sparkling ginger lemonade, you can mix with natural sparkling water, rather than simply purified water.

*Please note that sparkling water can be acidifying if carbonation is added and not natural

## 🍵 Food for Thought:

**Carbonated drinks are made from carbon dioxide—which is our waste/outbreath … something to think about.**

Remember the words of Raffi:

"All I really need, is a song in my heart, food in my belly and love in my family… and I need some clean water for drinking, and I need some clean air for breathing so I grow up big and strong and find my place where I belong."

Let us join in coming home, awakened and hungry for change. The medicine for our generation is in the plants, the microbes, ferments and our liberated re-membering, allowing ourselves to be wellsprings of joy, for the next seven generations unseen.

# References

1. Bush, Z. (2018). Biology base camp: Intrinsic Health series. intrinsichealthseries.com/biology-basecamp-webed-series/.

2. The Physicians for Responsible Medicine: pcrm.org.

3. Patel, J. (2000). Listen to your gut. Vancouver, BC: Caramel Publishing.

4. Conlon, M.A., & Bird, A.R. (2015). *The impact of diet and lifestyle on gut microbiota and human health nutrients.* 7(1), 17–44. http://doi.org/10.3390/nu7010017.

5. Johnson, A. (2017). *The microbiome and the gut-brain axis.* ThatSugarFilm.com.

6. Bush, Zach & Roll, Richie. (2018, March 18). *The Rich Roll Podcast—Zach Bush, M.D: GMOs,* glyphosate, and healing the gut.

7. University of North Carolina. (2016). *Benefits of mindfulness training.* Chapel Hill School of Medicine.

8. Kuo, Dr. Braden. (2015, June 18). *Study suggests that meditation and yoga may help symptoms of IBS and IBD.* Massachusetts General Hospital Research Institute.

9. Househam AM, Peterson CT, Mills PJ, Chopra D. (2017, Fall). The effects of stress and meditation on the immune system, human microbiota, and epigenetics. *advances in mind-body medicine.* 31(4):10-25.

10. Albenberg, L.G., Lewis, J.D., Wu, G.D. (2012). Food and the Gut Microbiota in Inflammatory Bowel Diseases: A Critical Connection.

(Abstract). *The National Center for Biotechnology Information.* (DOI: 10.1097/MOG.obo13e328354586f). Retrieved from www.ncbi.nlm.nih.gov/pmc/articles/PMC3822011/#!po=20.3704.

11. Cousens, G. (2003). *Rainbow green live—food cuisine.* Berkeley, CA: North Atlantic Books.

12. Mercola, J. (2016). *How your gut microbiome influences your mental and physical health.* Retrieved from: http://articles.mercola. com/sites/articles/archive/2016/01/07/ how-gut-microbiome-influences-health.aspx.

13. Mercola, J. (2016). *American gut project.* Retrieved from articles. mercola.com/sites/articles/archive/2016/03/13/nourishing-gut-bacteria.aspx.

14. Greenfield, R. and Levin, S. (2018, Aug. 11). Monsanto ordered to pay $289M as jury rules weedkiller caused man's cancer. *The Guardian.* Retrieved from: https://www.theguardian. com/business/2018/aug/10/monsanto-trial-cancer-dewayne-johnson-ruling.

15. McCumsey, S. (2019, Feb.). *An Essay on Pesticide Free Canada.* Personal Interview.

16. Phillips, J. (2019). Gardening For Peace. www.gardeningforpeace.com/.

17. Bush, Z., Gildea, J., Roberts, D., & Matavelli, L. (2019). The effects of ION*Bione dietary supplement on markers of intestinal permeability and immune system function in healthy subjects; a double-blind, placebo-controlled clinical trial. *Biomic sciences,* LLC, Charlottesville, VA.

18. Gottschall, E. (1994). *Breaking the vicious cycle*. New York, NY: Kirkton Press Limited.

19. Perlmutter, D. (2015) *BrainMaker*. New York, NY: Little, Brown and Company.

20. Gates, D. (1996). *The body ecology diet*. U.S.: Hay House Inc.

21. Miller, B. (Feb 04, 2017) I love you…actually I love your microbiome. *Huffpost*.

22. McClelland, D. (2015). *Irritable hearts: a PTSD love story*. New York: Flatiron Books.

23. Gershon, M. (1999). *The second brain*. New York: HarperCollins Publishers.

24. HeartMath Institute. *Activate the heart of humanity*. www.heartmath.org.

25. Pearsall, Paul. (1998). *The heart's code*. New York, NY: Broadway Books.

26. Batmanghelidj, F. (1992). *Your body's many cries for water*. London: The Tagman Press.

27. Junger, A. (2013). *Clean gut: The breakthrough plan for eliminating the root cause of disease and revolutionizing your health*. New York: HarperOne.

28. Chutkan, R. (2015). *The microbiome solution*. Penguin Random House. New York: NY.

29. Gracie, D.J., Williams, C.J.M., Sood, R., Mumtaz, S., Bholah, M.H., & Hamlin, J. 2017 Clinical gastroenterology and hepatology: *Negative effects on psychological health and quality of life of*

*genuine irritable bowel syndrome–type symptoms in patients with inflammatory bowel disease.*

30. Evans, J.M., Morris, L.S. & Marchesi, J.R. (2013) *The gut microbiome:* The Role of a Virtual Organ in the Endocrinology of the Host. *Journal of Endocrinology;* Society of Endocrinology.

31. Leonard, M. M., & Fasano, A. (2016). The microbiome as a possible target to prevent celiac disease. *Expert Review of Gastroenterology & Hepatology.* 10(5), 555–556. http://doi.org/10.1586/17474124.2016.1166954.

32. Mayer, E. (2016). The Mind/Gut Connection. HarperCollins Publishers, New York, NY.

33. Lyte, M., Cryan, J.F. (2014), Microbial endocrinology: The microbiota-gut-brain axis in health and disease. *Advances in Experimental Medicine and Biology.* 817, DOI 10.1007/978-1-4939-0897-4_1, Springer New York, NY.

34. Kellman, R. (2014). *The microbiome diet.* Boston, MA: First Da Capo Press.

35. Quigley, E. M. M. (2013). Gut bacteria in health and disease. *Gastroenterology & Hepatology*, PubMed Central. 9(9), 560–569.

36. Campbell-McBride, N. (2004). *Gut and psychology syndrome: Natural treatment of autism, ADHD, dyslexia, dyspraxia, depression and schizophrenia.* White River Junction: Medinform Publishing.

37. Schwenk, D. (2013). *Cultured food for life.* Carlsbad: Hay House Publishing Inc.

38. Bassler, B. (2009, Feb). How bacteria "talk." (Video file). Retrieved from www.ted.com/talks/bonnie_bassler_on_how_bacteria_communicate.

39. Perlmutter, D. (2013). Grain brain. New York, NY: Little, Brown and Company.

40. Yang B., Wei J., Ju, P., & Chen P.. (2019, April). Psychiatry Effects of Regulating Intestinal Microbiota on Anxiety Symptoms: A systematic review. *Journal of General Psychiatry*.

41. Forsythe P., Bienenstock J. & Kunze W.A. (2014). Vagal Pathways for microbiome-brain-gut axis communication. *Advanced Experimental Medical Biology*. 2014:817:115-33. doi: 10.1007/978-1-4939-0897-4_5.

42. Jockers, Dr. (2017). I*s Your Brain Making Enough GABA*,. Dr.Jockers.com.

43. Eckburg, P.B., Bik, E.M., Bernstein, C.N., Purdom, E., Dethlefsen, L., Sargent, M., Gill, S.R., et. al. Relman, D.A. (2005). *Diversity of the Human Intestinal Microbial Flora*. 308, (5728), 1635-1638 DOI: 10.1126/science.111059.

44. Lanphier, L. (2014). 11 *Foods highest in mycotoxins*. OAW Health, Oasis Advanced Wellness.

45. Young, R.O. (2009, Oct 5). *The history of monomorphism /pleomorphism*. Retrieved from phoreveryoung.wordpress.com/2009/10/05/the-history-of-monmorphismpleomorphism/.

46. Food & Beverage Company. (2017). *FoodMap.com*.

47. Rubin, J.S., Stanley, C.F. (2005, April 5). The maker's diet. Berkeley (first published March 12, 2004). ISBN 0425204138 (ISBN 13: 9780425204139).

48. Cousens, G. (2000). Depression free for life. New York, NY: HarperCollins Publishing.

49. Kim, Y.-S., Zheng, X.-B., & Shin. D.-H.. (2008). Growth inhibitory effects of kimchi (Korean traditional fermented vegetable product) against Bacillus cereus, Listeria Monocytogenes, and Staphylococcus aureus. J Food Prot. Feb; 71(2):325-32. PMID:18326182.

50. Cousens, G. (2000). Conscious eating. Berkeley, CA: North Atlantic Books.

51. Cousens, G. (1986). Spiritual nutrition. Boulder, CO: Cassandra Press.

52. Buettner, D. (2008). The blue zones. Washington, DC: the National Geographic Society.

53. Greger, M. FACLM Founder. NutritionFacts.org.

54. Glick-Bauer, M.,Yeh, M.C. (2014). *The health advantage of a vegan diet: exploring the gutmicrobiota connection.* The National Center for Biotechnology Information. (DOI: 10.3390 /null 114822). Retrieved from ww.ncbi.nlm.nih.gov/pmc/articles/ PMC4245565/#!po=1.19048.

55. Costantini, A.V., Mercola, J. (2008) *Does tainted milk cause disease?*

56. Rifkin, J. (1992). *Beyond beef.* New York, NY: Penguin Books. Smith, J. M. (2007).

57. Lee, M., Seo, D. J., Jeon, S. B., Ok, H. E. E., Jung, H., Choi, C.,

& Chun, H. S. (2016). Detection of foodborne pathogens and mycotoxins in eggs and chicken feeds from farms to retail markets. Korean Journal for Food Science of Animal Resources, 36(4), 463–468. http://doi.org/10.5851/kosfa.2016.36.4.463.

58. Blaser, M. (2015). *Missing microbes.* New York, NY: Pan Books Ltd.

59. Collins, S.M., Bercik, P., Park, A.J., Sinclair, D., et al. (2011) *The anxiolytic effect of Bifidobacterium longum* NCC3001 involves vagal pathways for gut-brain communication. *Neurogastroenterol Motil.* Dec. 23(12):1132-9.

60. Zeng, J., Li, Y.-Q., Zuo, X.-L., Zhen, Y.-B., Yang, J., Liu, C.-H.: (2008) Effect of active lactic acid bacteria on mucosal barrier function in patients with diarrhoea-predominant irritable bowel syndrome. *Aliment Pharmacol Ther.* 2008 Oct 15; 28(8):994-1002. Epub 2008 Jul 30. PMID: 18671775.

61. Young, R.O. (2009, Oct. 5). *The history of monomorphism/ pleomorphism.* Retrieved from phoreveryoung.wordpress. com/2009/10/05/the-history-of-monmorphismpleomorphism/.

62. Kelly, P.C., Lamont, J.T. (2017). *Patient education: Antibiotic-associated diarrhea caused by Clostridium difficile* (Beyond the Basics).

63. Haskey, N., & Gibson, D. L. (2017, Mar. 10). An examination of diet for the maintenance of remission in inflammatory bowel disease. *Nutrients.* I(3): 259. Published online. (doi: 10.3390/ nu9030259). PMCID: PMC5372922; PMID: 28287412.

64. Knox, N.C., Forbes, J.D., Van Domselaar, G., Bernstein, C.N. (2019) The gut microbiome as a target for IBD treatment: Are we there yet? *Curr Treat Options Gastroenterol.* Mar. 17(1):115-126. doi: 10.1007/s11938-019-00221-w.

65. Katz, S.E. (2002). *Wild fermentation: A do-it-yourself guide to cultural manipulation.* Portland, OR: Microcosm Publishing.

66. Challa, S. Dr. (2012). *Probiotics for dummies.* Hoboken, NJ: John Wiley and Sons, Inc.

67. Fiocchi, C. (1998) Inflammatory bowel disease: Etiology and pathogenesis by Claudio, Fiocchi, *Gastroenterology.*115, 185.

68. Rubin, J.(2018). *Garden of life:* www.gardenoflife.com.

69. Pinto-Sanchez MI, Hall GB, Ghajar K, et al. (2017) Probiotic *Bifidobacterium longum* NCC3001 reduces depression scores and alters brain activity: a pilot study in patients with irritable bowel syndrome. *Gastroenterology.* doi: 10.1053/j.gastro.2017.05.003.

70. *Human microbiome project.* https://hmpdacc.org/.

71. Zhou, L., Foster, J.A. (2015). Psychobiotics and the Gut–Brain Axis: In the Pursuit of Happiness. *Neuropsychiatric Disease and Treatment. 11,* 715–723. http://doi.org/10.2147/NDT.S61997.

72. Kattenburg, David. (2016, Feb. 19). Gut axis: Bacteria on the mind. *Green planet monitor.* Retrieved from: https://www.greenplanetmonitor.net/society-culture-arts/food/gut-brain-axis/.

73. Smith, J. (2014). *Genetic roulette.* www.youtube.com/watch?v=hAMlir8oprw.

74. David Crow, L.A. (2017). *Healing with botanical herbs: Virtual audio training.* Recorded January—April, 2017. The Shift Network.

75. Tuttle, W. (2005, 2016, Tenth edition). *World Peace Diet.* NY: Lantern Books.

# About the Author

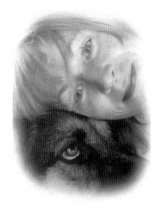

Tami S. Hay has spent three decades eating organic and has recovered from being very ill with Crohn's and colitis. In addition to witnessing many others heal in world-renowned wellness clinics, Tami has a master's degree in live food nutrition and has studied with some of the world's best integrative MDs. Her humility and her love as a Mother Bear have helped her turn her health around. She uses her daily research and integration to help her in teaching many other ways to eat food as medicine. She firmly believes that knowing there is hope and making changes can be easier than one thinks.

Tami lives with her dog, Bella. She shares her log country home with many friends, family, grandchildren, retreat participants, yogis, foodies, and plants and sprouts on the prairie near Edmonton, AB. She is in the process of writing her second book in this series, *EarthGut: Peace, Love, and Microbes for Foodies.*

*Tami Hay takes us deeper into the mind/body/spirit interface. Her journey to wholeness is inspiring with many helpful practices to support the body's healing journey.*

*~ Jini Patel Thompson, Director,*
*LISTEN TO YOUR GUT Enterprises Inc.*

Printed in Canada